metta

SENSES

WIDE

OPEN

loving kindness

skilled in good, wishing
to attain a state of calm, so
should one behave: able, upright,
perfectly upright, open-minded,
gentle, free from pride

SENSES

WIDE

OPEN

The Art and Practice of Living in Your Body

JOHANNA PUTNOI

FOREWARD BY ROBERT K. HALL

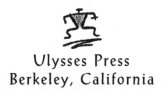

Ulysses Press
Berkeley, California

Published by: Ulysses Press
P.O. Box 3440
Berkeley, CA 94703-3440
www.ulyssespress.com

Library of Congress Catalog Card Number: 99-69195
ISBN: 1-56975-201-x

Printed in Canada by Transcontinental Printing

10 9 8 7 6 5 4 3 2 1

Editorial and production staff: Leslie Henriques, Steven Zah Schwartz, Claire Chun, David Wells, Lily Chou
Design: Leslie Henriques and Sarah Levin
Cover Illustration: "Poppies," SuperStock, Inc.

Distributed in the United States by Publishers Group West, in Canada by Raincoast Books, and in Great Britain and Europe by Airlift Book

I am a naked human
standing inside a mine of rubies,
clothed in red silk.
                        — RUMI

Man has no Body distinct from his Soul
for that calld Body is a portion of Soul
discerned by the five Senses,
the chief inlets of Soul in this age.

                    —WILLIAM BLAKE

To my parents,
Ruth and Martin Putnoi,
whose love created me and taught me
that my body was a precious thing

Contents

Foreword

The past century has been a time of great upheaveal in the world, in which the most appalling cruelty known by the human species has been perpetrated on ourselves and our home planet. Aggression, violence and destructive behavior have reached breathtaking magnitude. World wars, caused by the unbridled release of dark forces out of the human psyche, were fought with weapons of such massive power that one can only wonder at the miracle of our survival into a new millennium. There were times in our recent past when the total destruction of ourselves and our planet seemed a likely possibility. That danger is still very much with us.

Simultaneously, the past century has witnessed the emergence of an amazing upwelling of interest in self-awareness. As a species, we are currently being touched by a rising tide of curiosity and investigation into the nature of our own being. We have become seriously interested in discovering what "makes us tick."

The search for true self is becoming a legitimate task for ordinary intelligent people, no longer relegated just to the religious recluse or the isolated artist. Self-awareness training has found its way into the offices of large corporations, the halls of government, our churches, and into the lives of millions of ordinary citizens.

One aspect of this search for self-knowledge has been a growing interest in the ways we relate to our own living bodies. The human body is the vehicle for all our experience, personal and transpersonal. The life of the body is also the life of our collective society.

A wonderful outcome of our emerging interest in self-knowledge has been the gradual appearance, during the past 30 years, of a field called Somatics. This is a discipline that involves training the attention and focusing awareness on the actual experience of being an embodied organism. It is a systematic study of the life of the human body in present time, from the inside. It incorporates learning a number of methods for gaining direct awareness of bodily life that can lead to profound insight, and yet are essentially simple and available to anyone willing to make a commitment to practice them.

With expanded awareness of the body comes greater skill in living, working, and loving. Somatics offers the prospect of people becoming ever more compassionate toward each other and more adept at managing the hardships and mysteries of life as a human being.

Johanna Putnoi has given us, out of her many years of work and study, one of the first truly accessible guidebooks of Somatics. These pages are clear and artistic expressions of an incredibly exiting way to learn about ourselves. With great gratitude to Johanna, I invite you to enter into this study of life in the human body. It could change the way you view yourself and the world. It could even bring more compassion into the history of the human race, and we could all benefit from that.

Robert K. Hall, M.D.
Lomi School Foundation
Santa Rosa, California
and
Spirit Rock Meditation Center
Woodacre, California
February 2000

Acknowledgments

The process of writing this book has brought me great pleasure. It has taught me how to reach out for help in a way that allowed me to truly receive. I took a deep breath, shifted my attention to sensation, cleared my mind, and reached out from the heart. To my surprise and delight, I found abundance.

I have many to thank for supporting me in the process of bringing *Senses Wide Open* to life. Rose McDermott was the first to seriously suggest that I write a book, and has cheered me on tirelessly for seven years. This book would not exist without her.

Gabriele Hilberg and my Enneagram Group recognized that I was on to something one night. When Gabriele called the next day and generously offered to listen to me outline my ideas (not once, but week after week), it all just came together. Howard Teich showed me how my own narcissism was my greatest enemy as he encouraged me to write anyway. He sent me to Naomi Lucks, my trusty and inspired editor and friend. She sent me to Sheryl Fullerton, my no-nonsense, clear-minded agent, who found me a great publisher: Ulysses Press.

I am most grateful to my dear and patient friend Jane Ingalls for listening to me carry on and then editing the various incarnations of this book for spelling errors and split infinitives; to my extraordinary teaching partner and investment guru Robert Sanoff for keeping me honest and creditworthy; and to Larry Johnson for filling my heart with warmth and laughter while keeping my mind on the cutting edge of the virtual worlds.

Warm thanks to my cherished friends Jeanne Field, John Binder, Phoebe Larmore, Susan Kirk, Catherine Lemon, Peter Dergee, Elena Silverman, Jeanne Krois, Kristen Harrison, Carol Sanoff, Alice Moore, Lorraine Suter, Susan Hill, Ted and Margo, my sister, Sue Steck, my niece and nephew Jackie and Scott Cohen, and the spirit of Don McNeill for believing in me.

Thanks to Ray Riegert, Leslie Henriques, Steven Schwartz, Bryce Willett, Laura Dobb, Claire Chun, and all the folks at Ulysses; Phil Zimbardo, David Daniels, Mark Powelson, Janice Ross, Joan Minninger, Esalen Institute, and the Lomi Community: They all gave me their precious time and council when I asked. Thank you one and all.

I could not have attempted or completed this book without the guidance of my fierce and inspired teachers: Martha Graham, Bert Ross, Richard Patrick, David Leahy, Len Lye, Ivan Illich, Chloe Scott, Moshe Feldenkrais, Robert K. Hall, Richard Strozzi Heckler, Wendy Palmer, Michael Smith, Randy Cherner, Al Bauman, Emilie Conrad, Susan Harper, Heather Ogilvy, Helen Palmer, Carl Whitaker, Claudio Naranjo, and Howard Teich. Thank you for creating the ground on which to build my own life and work, for seeing me, for being exactly who you are.

Every one of my students and clients has contributed to my personal process and the evolution of this book. I have had the privilege to witness many struggles and victories over all these years. I have woven my observations into teaching stories that illustrate the possibilities for change that are catalyzed by learning to reference and respect the universal language of the body. It is my great hope that confidentiality has been maintained and that the stories will serve to help you in your search for connection and self-knowledge. Thank you for finding the courage to become all that you are.

Johanna Putnoi
Menlo Park, California
February 2000

Introduction

These days, when it is sometimes difficult to separate the actual from the virtual, please remember this: You reside in a miracle of nature, your very own human body.

For more than twenty years, I have worked to help all kinds of men and women develop a new awareness and respect for their body's natural intelligence, their mind's natural clarity, and their inborn capacity for pleasure. I have witnessed my own transformation and that of hundreds of others when they have been given permission to experience, explore, and enhance the ways the body moves, the mind thinks, and the emotions feel.

I am not talking here about becoming an athlete or a dancer, about "getting in shape" or "losing weight." I am talking about relearning how to access the remarkable natural intelligence of the body you were given to live in on the day you were born. The art and practice of living consciously in this body is so profound that once you begin, you will want to continue because you will understand how the ability to *feel* pleasure—combined with the study of conscious embodiment and a willingness to see things as they are—bring together the essential ingredients for leading a humane, honest, and joy-filled life.

This book is an invitation for you to come to your senses, to learn to understand your body's language, hear its innate wisdom, and regularly begin to experience your true feelings and sensations, your capacity to feel connected to the earth and all living things. The simple, meditation-like exercises presented here are the tools that help you do this. With discipline, effort, and a willingness to take responsibility for yourself and your actions, you will learn how to engage the body's wordless language, soften body armor, drop old defenses, and enjoy the world with senses wide open. You will begin to feel clear-minded, alive, delighted, and ready to explore this new-found realm that was there all the time.

My Story

Before you begin, I would like to share with you the story of how I first came to my senses and discovered how to feel more engaged with the world.

My mother said that I loved to dance from the very beginning— I was a happy, infectiously expressive child—and she enrolled me in ballet classes at the age of six. I couldn't get enough. The teacher said I was gifted. So when the United States Army ordered my family to move from Texas to New York City, Mom took me to audition at the prestigious Julliard School, where I was accepted. From there I went on to study modern dance with my first mentor, the innovative choreographer and dancer Martha Graham, until my father got orders and we had to move. Fortunately there were dance schools wherever we lived.

Like all dancers, I quickly learned to focus on what the mirror and the teacher told me. I became an expert at placing my attention on how my body looked and ignoring the messages that came from sensations like pain and pleasure. Little by little, I replaced my natural prepubescent movements with the trained but graceful and self-conscious gestures of a dancer. Pain in my body was something to ignore. It became, in fact, the banner of my commitment. After all, I was in the process of becoming every young girl's fantasy: "a beautiful dancer." I had no clue that I had entered the process of forgetting my body's natural language.

As fate would have it, I injured my right knee for the first time when I was a junior in high school. Even though the pain took my breath away, I continued to dance in my ballet company's performances and do all the other activities I loved until my knee lost strength and started aching all the time.

The x-rays my doctor father ordered showed nothing, and since it was time for me to go off to college, I apathetically stopped dancing. It never occurred to me that this might be connected to the general feeling of malaise that was invading my world.

In many ways I was excited to be away from home. I passionately joined the '60s revolution, marching against the war and experimenting with sex, art and rock and roll. But deep inside, I couldn't lose my sense that something important was missing.

Three years later, when my knee was interfering with regular walking, a doctor I consulted said that indeed there was something wrong. I needed surgery to remove a loose piece of cartilage from the fluid surrounding my knee. My father arranged for me to have the operation at a military hospital near New York University, where I was a college student. It was 1967 and I was nineteen years old.

I stayed in that hospital for two full weeks, without visitors, an innocent but privileged young woman surrounded by scores of wounded and dying soldiers shipped home from Vietnam. On television, I saw my college friends getting their heads beaten in as they demonstrated to close down the local Induction Center, while I shared my inadequate rehabilitation with boys who had lost their legs and arms and souls in Vietnam. I couldn't bear it. It wasn't difficult to see that my own pain was nothing compared to theirs. I kept "a stiff upper lip," as my family so patriotically advised, and wrestled with the realization that my marching and speaking out hadn't done much to stop the atrocities on either side.

The world I emerged to after that experience wasn't the same. I left the hospital numb, denying that the pain I had felt and witnessed was shattering. No one seemed to notice. Three months later I was hospitalized again. They had made a mistake during the first surgery and had to operate one more time. After two weeks I reentered my life with no rehab and less hope. The doctor said I could never dance again—that my knee was too weak to ever survive another injury, and I should get a desk job. That was it. I watched myself shrivel up and die inside. I had no guide to show me how to find the will to really live again.

Coming Home to My Body

In the fall of 1969 I traveled to California in search of myself. After many months on the road I met my next significant mentor, Chloe Scott, who recognized me as a dancer and invited me to join her dance troupe, Dymaxion Moving Company. Dymaxion was a wild mix of spirited nonconformists who were all blessed with perfectly imperfect bodies and proud of it.

Chloe showed me how I had replaced my natural way of moving with the vocabulary of ballet and modern dance. She introduced me to the beauty of the natural body in motion, got me performing again, and encouraged me to replace my fear with interest and spontaneity.

This provided me the direct experience of how my life thus far had been a product of mind over matter. My mind had forced my body to move in certain ways, whether it wanted to or not. To unblock my body I first had to educate myself about how the body was naturally designed to function, and then carefully coax my out-of-balance posture back to center. By consciously interrupting my destructive habit of whipping my body into shape, I was able to return my posture, along with the way I moved, to a more natural state. This was the way to real freedom, and I could feel the bonds loosening from deep inside my own skin.

In 1975 I traveled to the Naropa Institute in Boulder, Colorado, to formally study dance again. Naropa was on the cutting edge of education, one of the first new accredited institutions to offer degrees in Buddhist studies, in-depth psychology and the arts. In addition to the dance classes I had decided to take, I reluctantly signed up for an introduction to Gestalt Psychology on the recommendation of a friend who raved about the teacher, Robert K. Hall. I was reluctant because I suffered from the cultural bias that psychology was only for "crazy" people. I thought of it as stuffy and academic, and besides, I considered myself to be quite sane. To my great surprise, that teacher would become my next mentor.

Robert K. Hall was a psychiatrist, a poet, and one of the founders of the Lomi School. There was something about Robert's presence that awakened me—that gave me the courage to look deeper for the answers I was seeking. The fact that he was a medical doctor like my father made me pay attention to him in a different way.

Robert explained the philosophy of Gestalt psychology that he had learned from his mentor, Dr. Fritz Perls. He demonstrated clearly, as he worked with people during the class, that human neurosis is not just a mental concern: it takes up residence in body posture and emotional expression. The body couldn't change without the mind, and vice versa. I was moved by his willingness to simply hear a person's truth without judgment, to enable the person he was working with to see without blinders on. Class after class, I was amazed to realize how asleep people can be to what really ails them. They were ruled by something deep inside that kept them feeling confused and unhappy, doomed to keep repeating the same old behavior.

I was utterly captivated. I started to see myself in a new way. I learned what a powerful force the unconscious can be. I was more willing to admit how much I still suffered from my knee surgery, that I wasn't really happy, that I needed help in order to change. Best of all, I had that gut feeling. My body knew I had found my life path. I called to check out the Lomi School as soon as I returned to California.

Healing the Wounds

Since 1970, the Lomi School had been pioneering the integration of Western psychology and bodywork with Eastern spiritual disciplines. Its credo—that you can only touch another as deeply as you have allowed yourself to be touched—required students to work intimately and actively on their own issues of body, heart, and mind before they could become therapists. Its revolutionary approach would inspire many other similar schools, which today call the methods they practice and teach somatic work or body-centered therapy.

When I first visited the Lomi School I met a recent graduate named Randy. Upon telling him my tale of woe, the story of my botched knee surgery and all its repercussions, he told me he "specialized in knees." He said he could help me by manipulating my muscles and joints with the hands-on bodywork techniques he had learned at the school, and asked if I would like to make an appointment.

I will never forget that day. As this stranger worked with the muscles of my body, I could feel myself letting go. His touch felt great.

I had nothing to compare it to. He encouraged me to breathe deeply as he worked everywhere *except* my knee. I was sure he wasn't touching *that* because it was so ugly and damaged. I relaxed. And then, with no warning, he put his hands on my knee, and held it like it was a precious thing. In one moment I went from feeling fine to feeling deep grief. I began to sob uncontrollably. Embarrassed, I tried to stop. Randy asked me to roll over into the fetal position and covered me with a blanket. Rocking me gently, he said, "Don't try to explain, just let your tears flow, let your sounds sound. I'm right here—I'm not going anywhere."

I think I wept for forty minutes full out—for lost friends, for the wounded soldiers I'd met, for myself, and for all the suffering people in the world. I was submerged in a river of grief. I lost control of my mind and body. For the first time in my conscious life, I had the experience that someone could tolerate my pain. Randy didn't try to cajole me out of it. He didn't accuse me of indulging in self-pity. To my utter amazement, he encouraged me to experience my sorrow. Just as Robert had done for the people in the Gestalt class, Randy simply stayed there until I naturally emerged from this profound emotional release.

I felt as if a million pounds had been lifted off my chest.

He held me in his heartfelt gaze and said, "I am so sorry. You have suffered a great loss." He went on to tell me the truth. My knee, he said, would never be the same. It had been severely damaged and was indeed vulnerable to re-injury, but that wasn't my biggest problem. More serious was that the trauma induced by the surgery had caused me to vacate my knee, my leg, and my body in general, causing me to live in a constant state of disembodiment and fearful thinking. With a wisdom beyond his years, Randy said, "Until you grieve for what you have lost, you cannot discover what you have. The good news is that your knee works better than you think. If you place your attention on the actual sensations you are feeling, instead of on your fearful ideas about injuring it again, you will learn to distinguish between good pain and bad pain. You must learn to feel the knee you actually have. With time and effort, you can reeducate yourself. I can help you with this process." He did; and more than twenty years later, I am still dancing.

My knee injury has been one of my most powerful teachers. It has led me down a road that still compels and inspires me. What Randy said came true. The more I consulted the sensations in my body, the more I trusted myself. My knee recovered and the fear in my mind subsided. I felt like Dorothy entering Oz, when her black-and-white world changes into color. The domain of sensation became the focus of my exploration.

I enrolled at the Lomi School. I studied hands-on bodywork in combination with the Japanese martial art aikido, Vipassana meditation, Gestalt, and Reichian work. I learned how to feel and maintain a sense of balance or center in my body, heart, and mind. I learned how to protect myself through awareness. I learned what it meant to be present in the moment, as I actively engaged with my own experience. My resignation transformed into interest. I set about cultivating a relationship between my sensations, my feelings, and my thoughts. I was thirty-two years old. My body was well on the way to being fully mine.

Doing the Work: Humanity In Action

Much has happened since. I have had the good fortune to study with other innovative teachers in my field as I have continued teaching and learning, performing and dancing, honing my mind and heart and body. I continue to be amazed and inspired by people's stories, by the creativity and courage of the human spirit. "Life is not for sissies," they say, and that's for sure.

My story is a metaphor for a much greater issue: the cultural split between ideas and the language of the body. Our myths about the need to repress pleasure in order to lead a moral life, to pretend to be happy when we're not, to hold back emotions in order to appear strong, are the perverse results of this split. We are taught to suppress our natural instinctive responsiveness, and in the process we learn not to tell the truth, not to trust our instincts, not to touch. There are few places where we can witness authentic intimacy, where we can see our humanity in action.

I have been blessed with friends and teachers who have encouraged me to live from the essence of my nature, who have shown me that the key to tapping our inborn capacity to bond and to love one another is pleasure. Natural embodiment leads the way to what nourishes the soul, to the road that connects us to each other and to the larger body, earth's body. I write these words to pass that message along, to share with you what has filled my own life with meaning, inspiration and courage.

PART ONE

What Your Body Knows

CHAPTER 1

What Is Your Body Telling You?

Polish the heart, free the six senses and let them function without obstruction, and your entire body and soul will glow.

—MORIHEI UESHIBA

Right now, in this very moment: What is your body telling you?
Is your stomach tense with anxiety, or warm with relaxation?
Is your forehead furrowed in concentration, or are your eyes wide with wonder?
Are your feet happy in your shoes?
Is your breathing substantial yet tranquil?
Are you comfortable inside your own skin?
Are you looking out through your eyes, taking in sound through your ears, feeling the temperature with your skin, inhaling the scent of the air?
Are you living in your body right now?

Can you remember a time when your stomach knotted up in fear, your heart raced before an exciting challenge, you intuitively moved closer to a new love? Can you recall how your mind interpreted what your body felt? Did it berate you for being so weak (or cowardly or childish or out of control), ignore the sensation, and make your body do the exact *opposite* of what it knew was right?

"Trust your gut instinct" . . . "I knew in my heart it was the right thing to do" . . . "I just had a feeling" . . . Our language reflects

3

our understanding that the body has real wisdom and knowledge. Why, then, do we spend most of our time trying to override its signals?

The human body comes equipped with an innate ability to intuit real danger, and a brilliant physical response system that knows when to run and when to fight—even when we are actively not listening to the information we are receiving from our senses. The body also has the inborn ability to know when we are safe, to know who can nurture us emotionally, and to bond in love and support with others.

That's right: We are born with an innate instinct to survive and prosper, to love one another. One of the intrinsic ingredients that allows us to thrive is the experience of pleasure. However, when we are not actively listening to the information we are receiving from our senses, when we are taught that the language of the body will get us into trouble, it is much more difficult to respond naturally, to bond in long-lasting satisfying relationships with others.

Feeling fully alive means engaging life with our senses and instincts wide open. Touch is the mother of the senses. It is born with the oldest, largest, and most sensitive of our organs, the skin. Ashley Montagu, in *Touching,* his wonderful book about the significance of the skin, says: "The skin is the mirror of the organism's functioning; its color, texture, dryness, and every one of its other aspects, reflect our state of being, psychological as well as physiological. We blanch with fear and turn red with embarrassment. Our skin tingles with excitement and feels numb with shock; it is a mirror of our passions and emotions."

The skin covers our entire body. It is the foundation on which all the other senses are based. Our skin is the interface between our nervous system and the environment in which we live. It connects the outside to our insides, and vice versa. Neuro-anthropologist André Virél says, "Our skin is a mirror endowed with properties even more wonderful than those of a magic looking glass."

The skin is an essential player in the conundrum of our existence, in our striving for radiant well-being and connection to all things. It is our skin that allows us to differentiate between sandpaper and marble, glass and water, hot and cold, pain and pleasure. When we add taste, smell, sight, and hearing to this biological equation, a magnificent symphony of feeling and sensation informs our experience. Without our senses we are like stick figures—without sense and sensibility, forever ensnared in the modern disease of cerebral reasoning.

Unfortunately, most of us learn at an early age that the life of the mind is the real life, the important life, the body's high commander. The fullness of life—sensation and emotion—are subjugated to what we think at any given moment. Without the full palette of sensual input, life is reduced to a monochromatic dimension that has little room for the colors and sounds and smells and tastes and sensations that enable us to experience genuine pleasure and delight.

Living with senses wide open—learning to listen to the innate language of the body with conscious awareness—is what this book is about.

The Language of the Body

When we are warm and safe and well-nourished, our muscles relax, our blood flows easily, and we feel a sense of well-being or authentic pleasure. When we are in danger, cold and hungry, we feel anxiety and fear. Our muscles tense up, our breathing gets shallow, and we get ready to run.

I call this intrinsic intelligence *natural embodiment*. We are naturally embodied when we can experience sensate pleasure on a regular nonsexual basis, when we can deeply relax into ourselves, when we can give freely to other people and receive from them easily, when we know the difference between hedonism and authentic pleasure.

Animals move freely, effortlessly. They drop down for a nap when they are tired, they eat when they are hungry. We envy this natural state, but it is not ours. Being human means we have self-awareness. As human beings we are born with the unique ability to consciously observe and control our own behavior. Sometimes this is what gets us into trouble. Sometimes our minds don't like what we see, or we fear what might happen and we override our bodies' messages. Yet this awareness can also work to our benefit: We can train ourselves to move and think and hear and see and feel in ways that bring the world to life in infinite, unseen detail, much as a trained violinist can make a violin sing in tones that are beyond the reach of the student.

Conscious awareness naturally includes the language of the body. It helps us respond more honestly to what is happening in the moment. It helps us filter out neurotic thinking in favor of natural embodiment. I know this is true because I see it every day.

For more than twenty years I have worked with hundreds of disenfranchised human beings who are in search of their bodies and don't know it. Like most of us, they suffer terribly from our culture's mixed messages. Many of them are full of guilt and shame, trying unsuccessfully to reason their way through life. They have very little real information about the nature and function of their bodies' desires, illnesses, knee-jerk behaviors, and pleasures. Instead, their minds have developed elaborate mythologies about what might happen if they let go and allow their bodies to speak to them. Surely, they think, they would lose control sexually, or hurt themselves, or do something they would regret. Their fears are deep and powerful and keep them in the dark about how the body actually works. Paradoxically, they take their health for granted.

When we feel sick, we passively let the doctor tell us about our afflictions and follow medical directions without question. Our ignorance is staggering.

The last two decades of the twentieth century have been characterized by a frantic search for self-improvement and purification: We join programs to give up smoking, drinking, and drugs. We train our bodies in gyms. We eat carefully controlled diets to starve our bodies into submission. We buy books on how to improve our sex lives. We live hard and fast, seeking excitement, and then recover by meditating on inner peace, chasing out-of-body experiences and longing for a less corporeal world. We spend billions of dollars on diet, fitness, entertainment, and religion, and we are still not satisfied.

The simple truth is this: In seeking to perfect our bodies, tire them out, or escape them altogether, we have forgotten a fundamental point. We can't go anywhere without them, even though we try. The body matters. It's a resource, not an object to whip into shape. It is you.

Having a body is what being a human is all about.

Sarah's Story:
Learning to Listen to the Body's Language

Sarah's story is a good example of what can happen when you don't understand your body's language, and how you can begin to reconnect with its messages. A gregarious, attractive, thirty-six-year-old mother of three, Sarah had been suffering from nausea, headaches, intestinal pain, heart palpitations, and other disturbing physical symptoms for some time. When she finally consulted a doctor, he suggested she needed surgery to remove her gallbladder. When the lab tests showed gallstones, she reluctantly agreed.

As fate would have it, this simple surgical procedure went awry. Instead of a few days in the hospital, as the doctor had promised, Sarah had to spend one week away from her family and three more recovering at home in bed. Yet even after she was declared healed by her doctor, she continued to feel the same symptoms as before. Her surgeon said it was impossible—the gallbladder was out, so the symptoms must be in her head. Not long after that, Sarah began having severe anxiety attacks—nausea, intestinal pain, heart palpitations, and "a feeling of dread in the pit of her stomach"—that prompted her to schedule an appointment to see me.

In our phone interview, Sarah told me only that she "needed help in managing her stress." Early in our first stress-reduction session, I was surprised when Sarah showed me the angry red scar on her upper abdomen. And I was confounded when she dismissed it as "Oh, just some gallbladder surgery."

Clearly, she was in denial about the toll that the surgery had taken on her. Her overall tension, together with her vague answers about her physical sensations, led me to wonder if her symptoms had deeper roots. Had this gallbladder incident triggered a body memory of some other major trauma?

I recommended that Sarah attend my movement meditation classes. These classes are designed to acquaint participants with the difference between the discomfort caused when the mind whips the body into shape and the exquisite tones of sensation that come when we allow our bodies to move naturally.

When she tried these exercises for the first time, Sarah reported she felt only fear and sadness. She told me that as far back as she could remember, fear had been her constant companion. With this feeling so fresh in her system, she finally told me the story of her mother's tragic and painful fight with multiple sclerosis. The oldest child of three, Sarah was forced to play the little mother from an early age. She took her burden seriously, never finding the time and space to play like an ordinary kid. She was constantly afraid that something would go wrong, continually aware of how helpless she was, and sadly deprived of the loving touch that comes with healthy mothering.

When we are denied the comfort and feeling of safety that comes from regularly being held and cuddled by our parents, we often fail to develop our sensate awareness; an unpredictable, traumatic childhood can cause a person to replace direct body feedback, or sensation, with fearful thinking. I described how this common defense mechanism helped Sarah avoid the emotional pain of not having a healthy mom. She had trained herself to think of something else while she cared for her mother. This kept her separated not only from her emotional pain, but from her bodily life, a state that had come to feel normal after thirty years.

Now she was playing the same game but with a different twist. She couldn't stop thinking fearful thoughts even though she was well, and she would work herself up into an anxiety attack that made her feel crazy.

Over the weeks we worked together, Sarah began to understand the connection between her past and her present state of obsessive worry. Her excessive fears that the surgery hadn't been effective— that some of the botched procedures were the cause of her ongoing gallbladder symptoms, that the doctors were lying to her about the outcome—now made perfect sense. Her mind had taken control because she hadn't developed much of a relationship to the pleasure response. Instead of allowing herself to experience her actual physical sensations, over-thinking had caused her to feel bodily pain that mimicked gallbladder distress.

Now, however, she was inspired to replace her old method of seeing everything through the lens of her mind with a more balanced perception. Gradually, she began to let go of old habits and replace them with deeper ways of perceiving her world. For example, she told me that now when she starts to worry an ordinary event into a worst-case scenario, she says to herself, "Hold on a minute, Sarah. Before you get too carried away, take a deep breath and feel your body. Look around you. Can you see any actual danger coming toward you? Do you feel any pain in your body? Are you hungry? Keep breathing. Feels to me like we are safe. Please stop worrying and get on with the real work of the day."

Sarah said now that she understands the anatomy of her anxiety attacks, she can interrupt them before they take hold completely. Because they are no longer a mystery, she is far less tortured by the worried fantasies of her habitually fearful mind.

Learning to respect and listen to the language of the body changed Sarah's life for the better in many surprising ways. She learned to differentiate fearful thoughts that trigger anxiety attacks and body pain from genuine body sensations. When her anxiety attacks disappeared, Sarah's gallbladder symptoms stopped. For the first time in her life, she was able to feel comfortable in her own body.

And there was another bonus. Once Sarah understood where her overreliance on mind over matter had come from, her entire attitude changed. In the past she had been too suspicious of life to be open to the sensations her body was sending her, and feeling pleasure seemed foreign and even dangerous. She found she was not only willing to go deeper, but was excited about exploring her inborn ability to feel sensation and become fluent in the language of the body.

The results were impressive. Sarah no longer had to rely on the visual pleasure of the mind alone. She was able to experience the comfort induced by the feeling of authentic pleasure. With sparkling eyes, she recounted how her new-found experience of natural embodiment was enhancing her relationships with her children. She was more comfortable holding them close. She was better able to comfort them when they cried because she knew how to use her body to do so. She knew firsthand the difference between touch that comforts and touch that pushes away or invades.

This understanding also transformed her sexual and emotional life with her husband. She now knew how to relax and allow her whole self to respond more naturally. When she mentioned this to me, I told her the best kept secret of stress reduction is pleasure induction!

Let Your Body Be Your Teacher

Right now, stop reading and try the following exercise.

Try This Now:

> Take this moment to stretch your arm out in front of you.
>
> Look at your arm with your eyes.
>
> What do you see?
>
> When I look at my own arm, my mind and eyes tell me that my arm is solid. I see that it is made of completely different stuff than the space around it. I can easily see where my arm ends and space begins. Is that true for you too?

That is the truth of the eyes. Here is another truth: Everything—animate and inanimate—is moving and connected. In the body, everything is connected by the connective tissue. On the planet, everything is connected by shared atoms and molecules. Everything is infinitely recycled; we pass in and out of one another at every moment. Truly, there is nothing new under the sun: The water in your coffee cup this morning might once have been the sweat on King Tut's brow.

History tells us that some of our ancestors regarded the body and the earth as teachers. Morris Berman, the renowned scientific historian and author, addresses this in his groundbreaking book, *Coming to Our Senses:*

> Storytellers make an assumption that historians rarely do, namely that human beings are not rational, that they cannot be understood in terms of "objective" analysis, and that their deepest and most significant experiences are lived on a level that is largely invisible, a shadowy re-

gion where the mind and body move in and out of each other in an infinite number of elusive combinations, and that can only be evoked through allusion, feeling tone, rhetoric, and "resonance."

Try This Now:

Read the following instructions and then try the exercise. Better yet, have someone read them to you.

> Close your eyes.
>
> Stretch your arm out in front of you.
>
> Sense your arm, don't visualize it.
>
> Can you perceive your arm without using your eyes to tell you that it is there?
>
> Perhaps you feel only the weight of it.
>
> Perhaps you can only feel your shoulder and fingers, with a big black hole in between.
>
> In the domain of sensation, your arm becomes a completely different something.
>
> What do you feel?

If the first thing you feel is pain in your shoulder from holding your arm out, lower it to a more comfortable position. Pain is not the primary barometer here, normal sensation is.

Try This Now:

> Move your arm slowly for some minutes, as if it were under water.
>
> Allow your shoulder, elbow, wrist, and fingers to swim.
>
> Let your arm move you.

> Keep bringing your attention back to the simple feelings of sensation in your arm.
>
> Please, don't be seduced by thinking.
>
> Now stop.
>
> Stretch your arm out in front of you again.
>
> Notice if you now have some new sensate information about your arm.
>
> Is there some heat, or some tingling, or some pulsing moving throughout your entire arm? Do you have a whole arm in your sensate world now?

You can apply this simple exercise to other parts of your body. The more you move in this way, the deeper your attention gets, the wider the spectrum of sensations becomes. Your body awakens, muscles relax, awareness opens to new horizons.

Your Body Is Intelligent

As your eyes settle in on this page and begin to gobble up these words to place them in your mind, and as your mind begins to consider them, remember: At this very moment you also have a body.

Your body is a profoundly intelligent, biologically programmed miracle of nature that can translate the dreams of your mind into reality.

Your body has the capacity to feel an infinite spectrum of sensations and emotions.

Your body comes equipped with the instinct to bond, the ability to love. It offers you the chance to experience love and pleasure exquisitely intertwined in the mysterious, erotic domain of sensation.

Your body has the wisdom and ability to let you know when you are in danger, to tell you when you have met a kindred spirit, to tell you when it needs nourishment, to let you know it is time to rest.

At your most complete, you are a living, breathing, fully dimensional being, inhabiting your body with awareness. Your heart, mind, and spirit are fully integrated, expressing themselves through your body. This integration is the natural embodiment that is your birthright. But if you are like most people today, you are inhabiting only one or at best two narrow segments of your multidimensional self.

Strange as it may sound, most of us do not truly inhabit our own body. Some of us live primarily in the negative portion of the mental realm, fearful and tentative or filled with grandiose fantasies, thinking the world into some sort of sense. Some of us live primarily in the negative portion of the emotional realm, sinking into a swamp of despair or suddenly flying high, overdramatizing each event in order to feel intensely. Some of us live primarily in the negative portion of the physical realm, habitually angry at our aches and pains, at the uncomfortable physical world around us—that is irritatingly too hot, too cold, too smoky, too noisy, too dirty—or passive-aggressively leaving the modern world behind in favor of a life of pleasure-seeking on the ski slopes or the ocean waves, unable to separate indolence from natural instinct and clear-mindedness.

When we stand just outside ourselves in this way, our humanity lives somewhere else and our body feels empty and separate—a machine we can fix when it breaks down, replacing parts as needed. We judge this body mercilessly against a media-fed ideal—"working it out" with repetitive exercises that deny the organic cellular workings of our nature, starving it into submission with diets, deadening it with painkillers. We are disconnected from the earth and the human community, unable to touch ourselves or others on the deepest levels.

You don't have to read a book in order to learn how to walk or talk. You don't have to be told something is funny in order to break into spontaneous laughter. Sometimes you understand a thing is true intuitively, even though you have never learned it before. Does that seem strange?

Your body is a marvelous container for your self. At this very moment, within your body, a heart is pumping blood; involuntary muscles are working your liver, stomach, intestines, and lungs; a system of nerves far more complex than the electrical wiring in your house is helping you feel; and a column of vertebral bones that fit together perfectly provide strength and flexibility at the same time. Your body is an intelligent being in its own right, and when it is allowed to function in accordance with its brilliant natural design, you can trust it to do its job.

Try This Now:

> Come back to your felt body for a moment, to the world of sensations.
>
> Can you feel the weight of yourself sinking into the chair?
>
> Can you feel the air against your cheek, the texture of your clothes on your skin?
>
> Take a full, deep breath into your lungs.
>
> Feel the sensation.
>
> Relax your jaw, exhale through your mouth, and let your tension go.
>
> I promise all the things you have to think about will wait for you, so why not take a minute just to be here?
>
> Be here with yourself.

CHAPTER 2

Opening Your Senses

*[Our civilization] equates literacy with literature
. . . with the printed text; it does not consciously
understand that there is such a thing as body
literacy.*

— MORRIS BERMAN,
COMING TO OUR SENSES

Look around you: What do you see?
Listen: What do you hear?
Be aware of your skin: What does it feel?
Inside your mouth: What is the taste?
Inhaling: What do you smell?

There are as many tones of sensation as there are tones of sound
or hues of color. A magnificent symphony of sensation is playing in
your body right now. You can enjoy this body music when you learn
to allow your attention to drop from your mind into your body, expanding your awareness into every cell.

You were born to take in information from the world in order to
make sense of your place in it. You eat food in order to keep your
body alive. In the same way, each of your senses can work like a
mouth, taking different kinds of information into your body to nurture it. You have the innate ability to swallow down into your very

insides the most precious experiences that each of the senses provide. You have the capacity to receive.

We have come to believe that what we see with our eyes is most real because we think it is objective. I am talking here about the division between psyche and soma, that age-old dilemma that pits ecstatic experience against moral law and ultimately fosters a deep sense of separation.

Unfortunately, in the West we generally learn at an early age to separate the language of the body from the thoughts of the mind, and then to believe the mind: "I'm from Missouri—show me." "I only believe what I see with my own two eyes." This really means "I only believe the interpretation my mind gives me after it digests the information I received through my eyes."

But seeing with the eyes is not the only way to know the world. We have five physical senses—sight, hearing, taste, smell, and touch —as well as a latent intuitive sense. The senses are a primary part of human communication. They provide an experiential feedback system that informs us about ourselves and the intentions of those around us. Un-self-conscious responsiveness lives in the realm of the senses. When we add the intention of being present to our sensate experience, moment by moment, we can learn how to shift our awareness from thinking to sensation and feel how deeply healing natural embodiment is.

When we bring awareness to our senses and our instincts, we discover what it means to be human. But our humanity is forced underground when we denigrate the body as the prisoner of the soul— when we label it "dangerous," "dirty," "sinful," "too fat," "too thin," "ugly," "great looking," or "plain." This is the point of view that encourages us to manipulate our bodies like objects that need to be exercised and disciplined. Sadly, few of us have learned to respectfully include the authentic natural intelligence of the body as a fundamental source of our experience.

If we are not attentive, language takes the place of experiencing. "Tree," we say, and pass by without taking in the smell of the leaves, the texture of the bark, the hugeness of this living thing that stands for years without needing to remember itself. "Da Vinci," we say, and pass by without noticing the enigmatic images on the canvas or whether there is meaning for us here. "Police officer," we say, as we suck in our breath and hurry by without noticing if he or she is on duty, smiling, tired, or looking for offenders.

Language tends to separate us from bodily life. Try seeing without naming. Hearing without naming. Sensing without naming. When we extend what the Buddhists call unconditional regard to another, body to body, reality is no longer informed so much by ego. We enter a place where time slows down, where colors and scents affect us in a different way. This is the world below rational thought. In this place our gut tells us that we are all made of the same stuff.

Allow the World to Touch You, and You Will Touch the World

Healthy, normal people love to be touched, crave to be touched. Children leap into their parents' laps for comforting touch and assurance. The touch of a loved one, or even a caring stranger, soothes fear and grief. If you have forgotten that, watch how cats and dogs snuggle up and demand affection from their human friends.

Touch is fundamental to our experience of pleasure. The neuropsychologist James W. Prescott concluded from his research in the 1970s that certain sensory experiences and deprivations during early childhood development create a neuropsychological disposition for either violence-seeking or pleasure-seeking behavior later in life. According to Prescott, "The deprivation of body touch, contact, and movement are the basic causes of a number of emotional disturbances which include depressive and autistic behaviors, hyperactivity, sexual aberration, drug abuse, violence, and aggression." Ashley Montagu says, "When we speak of 'keeping in touch' we know whereof we speak, that it is not a mere metaphor but a consummation much to be desired."

We are in an ancient struggle between the external and the internal. We are caught in a painful split between mind and body. We have been taught to believe that the body is the bad guy, the one who sins, looks imperfect, and ultimately dies, taking us with it. We are taught to value our thoughts over our instincts and emotions, to value our objective scholarly investigation over our subjective direct experience. We think of our senses as tricksters, of the needs of the body as dangerous. We learn that only the rational mind has the ability to understand the "real" truth.

When you touch without thinking, your senses reveal a different reality. Touch is not just something you do with your hands and feel through your fingers. Sensation is a physical feeling evoked by any of the five senses. What you feel at any given time, what you remember about a given situation is often bound up with your sense of touch—"It was so cold that winter!" "My hands were like sandpaper after we remodeled the bathroom." "I love to wrap up in my warm, soft down comforter." In India they make paintings of humans with eyes all over the body, acknowledging the truth that it is possible to perceive the world not only with the eyes, but with the body. Through touch.

Both touch and touching animate the body's wordless language. There are many ways to touch. Deep massage of the muscles helps to release tension and cultivate relaxation. Soft touch enlivens the tissues and makes you feel more awake. You can learn to play the body like you can learn to play a musical instrument.

What a shame that we are never taught how to touch, that we recognize abuse in parents who strike their children, but fail to see abuse in parents who never touch their children. Our fear that "touch leads to inappropriate sex" has left us more afraid to touch and to be touched than interested in the nature of informed touch.

Try This With A Partner:

If you don't have a partner to do this exercise with, you can do it with your own body.

> Ask your partner to lie down face up, on a
> comfortable mat on the floor.

> Take a moment for both of you to quiet your mind
> and relax your body.

> Remember the exercise you did earlier with your arm.

Place your hand on your partner's back.

Simply feel the sensation of flesh on flesh.

Feel the expansion of the muscles between the ribs
during inhalation.

Feel the warmth building in your hand.

Imagine that your hand is part of your partner's body.

Imagine that this is water touching water.

Your hand takes the sensation in.

Your hand sees.

Your hand swallows the sensation like a mouth and
your whole being is warmed.

When you feel complete, ask your partner to sit up. Have a conversation about what this was like for each of you.

Hear Sound with Every Fiber of Your Body

Sound is not merely noise you hear through your ears: It is vibration that works on every part of your body. You can hear sound vibrations with your bones. You can feel the deep resonance of a drum in your chest, echoing your heartbeat. A note sung at the right vibration can shatter glass. Muscles are soothed by the music of violins or made tense by the wail of sirens. The sound of waves breaking on the sand can lull you to sleep.

Our ears are amazing mechanisms. Like our eyes, they are a distance sense. They tell us more about what is going on outside of us than inside of us. We tend to believe what we hear, just as we believe what we see.

Our ears allow us to take in the world around us in extraordinary ways. They provide us the ability to listen to the underlying tone that surrounds the words and sounds that come to us. We can hear the bass line underneath the melody, the violins that come in over the vocals. Our ears alert us to danger and soothe us to sleep.

When we hear the voice of a beloved, the body softens and is filled with feeling. When we hear a gunshot, the body tenses and drops to the ground without thinking. Hearing is both essential to survival and a doorway to pleasure.

Your ears receive and process sound so that you can swallow it down into the deepest regions of your insides, so that your skin can feel and your eyes can know better what they see. You hear with every fiber of your body.

Try This Now:

> Relax and take a deep breath.
>
> Hum a deep, low, "mmm" sound.
>
> As you do, feel the "mmm" go deep into your body.
>
> Can you feel the inside of your skull vibrating?
>
> Let these vibrations move down into the rest of your body "container"and enliven your tissues like a pond reed in the wind.

Try This Now, or Later:

> Listen to your favorite symphony.
>
> Don't think.
>
> Let the sounds enter your body.
>
> Let your muscles bathe in glorious resonance.

Try This with a Partner:

> Choose a piece of music you both like.
>
> Sit down in a chair facing your partner.
>
> Close your eyes, and take a deep, relaxing breath.
>
> Feel your back against the chair, your feet on the floor.

> Make yourself available to your partner and to the
> sounds you are about to hear.
>
> Open your ears and your heart.
>
> Receive the music without thinking.
>
> Let it enter you, move through you, pleasure you.

When the music is over, sit in silence together for a few minutes.
When you are ready, have a conversation about how you are feeling
now, about your impressions during the listening, about whatever
moves you.

Be Informed by Smell

Dogs live in a world made up almost entirely of scent, which they
can interpret in astounding detail. They know who passed by an hour
ago, they know you recently had contact with a cat, they know which
green tennis ball belongs to them. All because they are able to perceive each unique scent.

Humans do not have this highly developed olfactory sense, so
try as we might, we cannot live in world of scent like dogs do. Yet—
consciously and unconsciously—what we smell provides powerful
information. The smell of smoke alerts your other senses to prepare
to fight a fire or run. An unpleasant smell tells us something has
spoiled. Through the perfume of pheromones, your sense of smell
recognizes your lover before your eyes do. The scent of jasmine cools.
The scent of musk evokes the erotic. There is nothing precisely like
the awakening scent of lightning and thunder, or a flower-scented
moonlight night in the tropics.

Try This Now:

> Close your eyes and simply breathe.
>
> What do you know right now because of your sense
> of smell?
>
> Allow your nostrils to gently open and take
> nourishment from the air.

Can you taste smell?

Does smell trigger feelings? Memories? Movements?

Feel the sensation of breath as it enters your nose.

Can you feel this dark cavity inside your skull?

Does smell heighten sensation in other parts of
your body?

Taste Everything

Smell evokes taste: the two are irrevocably connected. If you lose your ability to smell, you also lose your ability to taste. Think what colors would leave your world without taste!

Your tongue is covered with taste buds, each one tasting something slightly different. Bitter, sweet, sour, tart, tangy, bland, noxious . . . the hues of taste are wonderful and awful. Taste warns you when the food is dangerous and soothes you when it is delicious. Put a little sugar on different parts of your tongue. Does it still taste as sweet?

Feel your tongue in your mouth. Run it over your teeth and gums.

Put something you love the taste of in your mouth and chew it slowly and carefully. Savor it fully and notice how taste enhances sensation. See with your mouth.

Try This Now or When the Time is Right:

Take a breath and get in your body.

Prepare your favorite food in silence.

Allow the aromas to enter your body through
your nostrils.

Notice how the smell of cooking changes the taste
and color of the food.

When your food is prepared, sit down and take a
deep breath.

Feel your feet on the floor and your back against the
   chair.

Now, place your attention inside your mouth.

Relax your tongue and jaw.

Feel the act of reaching for the food, lifting your fork
   or hand to your mouth.

Taste the food.

Now chew.

What does chewing do to taste?

Keep this deliciousness in your mouth for a while.

Chew it as if it were a precious thing, the elixir
   of life.

Chew it as if you have no need for anything more.

Just be present to the taste without thought.

Now swallow and be still for a minute.

Listen to what your body tells you.

Listen to what taste tells your body.

See Without Naming

Your eyes are hooked to thought in a way that no other sense is.
This is because they have a direct line into the brain through the
optic nerve. All the information you take in through your eyes goes
directly to your brain for interpretation. How you interpret that information depends on cultural bias, your upbringing, on your unconscious habits and expectations.

Because of this close connection, it's easy to become eye-thinking
dominant. We get caught in the habit of seeing to think rather than
seeing to *see*. That's why it is especially important to practice seeing
without naming. Seeing is entirely different when we don't attach a
name to what is seen.

Try This Now:

> Close your eyes and relax the surrounding muscles.
>
> Open your eyes and let them settle on a flower.
>
> Imagine that your eyes are a mouth.
>
> Swallow down into your body only what you
>   love to see.
>
> Take these images into your tissues.
>
> Let them swim in your blood.
>
> This is the key to your empathic sense—your
>   connection to all things.

When you look into the face of a friend, can you sense/feel where your seeing originates from? Do you feel the sensation of your eyes in your own head seeing out, or does it feel as if your vision begins on your friend's face—as if your eyes are housed in what it is you see?

You can play with how you choose to see and how you want to process it. You can use your eye muscles to hold your eyes still. This works to keep what you see outside yourself and separate. (You do this automatically when you are angry or threatened by someone or something.) You can soften the muscles around the eyes to let what you see in.

Try This Now:

> Think of your eyes as a telescope.
>
> Lengthen the lens, and what's seen becomes
>   foreground.
>
> You might even mistake what you see for part of
>   yourself.
>
> Shorten the lens and you bring your vision back into
>   your head.
>
> Your eyes are more like a window now.
>
> You feel as if you are inside yourself, looking out.

This is an interesting experiment to try with someone you feel enmeshed with—a parent or spouse, a baby or a lover. Sometimes it is important to feel separate and safe. Other times blending is the preferred choice. How nice to have a choice!

Try This Next:

>Sit comfortably in a chair. Place one hand on your chest, the other in your belly.

>Feel the warmth of your own hands radiating into your body.

>Take in a breath and let your back sink into the chair, your feet into the floor.

>Relax your eyes.

>Feel the space around you, the weight of gravity coming down through your bones and muscles.

>Now try the eye exercise again.

>Living in your body really is a palpable experience, isn't it?

CHAPTER 3

Minding the Body: How Your Posture Tells Your Story

The life of the body is our real life, the only life we have.

— MORRIS BERMAN,
COMING TO OUR SENSES

One night I was watching a nature documentary about sea lions on TV. The commentator said, "Look at the cute, mischievous sea lions on the rocks. Watch them diving into the waves." Cut to an underwater camera. "Here they are swimming and playing and hunting."

He called each sea lion by a name, but they all looked the same to me. Then I had this funny thought. What if this documentary was about *Homo sapiens*—you know, us humans?

Take two: "Look at the humans sitting on the rocks. Omigod, they're naked. Get the children out of the TV room!"

Few of us have ever seen an average adult male or female human (besides, perhaps, our mate) naked and moving naturally. We have little concept of what the body would be like if we lived in it un-self-consciously. Living with senses wide open means experiencing sensate pleasure regularly, nonsexually, and nonintellectually. It means being able to find and maintain our sense of center, even when the going gets rough. And it means being able to deeply relax—with or without our clothes on!

Our Body Armor Protects Us From—What?

We spend twenty-four hours a day in our bodies—it's a life sentence. Yet most people have little experience of the body simply as it *is*. We love to watch animals in their natural habitat, and we marvel at tribal peoples in their native surroundings, but we cannot allow our "civilized" selves to be seen naked and unadorned. Instead, we have come to associate nudity with pornography and shameful, cheap sex. Our nude people seem to live only in magazines like *Playboy* or *Playgirl* or on the Internet. These surgically enhanced, airbrushed young women and men beckon to us, titillating and frustrating us at the same time. They leave us feeling inferior of body, with superiority of mind as the booby prize.

We really don't know what else to do with the body, so we dress it up, hoping that clothing really does "make the man (or woman)." We may clothe our nakedness in garishly revealing clothing, or in uncomfortable clothing that inhibits movement. Whichever mode we choose, the result is the same: We feel alienated, uncomfortable, and unwelcome in our own body-home.

The messages we get from the outside world often make us feel dissatisfied with what we have. We pour far too much energy into lamenting our flaws—into feeling beaten and helpless, or angry and envious, or anxious and cursed.

This shame and discomfort doesn't just stay in our mind. It is translated by our body into holding patterns that create unnatural muscle tensions and postures called *body armor*. We hold our stomachs in so we'll seem slimmer or taller. We stuff our mobile and intelligent feet into tight, stylish shoes and end up causing pain and deformities. We slump into our shame, attempting to hide our bad features, our height, our sexuality, our excitement. Or we puff up into our narcissistic pride, exaggerating our natural beauty. But the truth is that most of us feel like we got the wrong body when God was doling them out. "If only I had gotten Cindy Crawford's (or Brad Pitt's) face and body . . . *then I would be happy!*"

The body and the being inside—you—were originally designed to work seamlessly together. One "body-self" moving naturally through the world. But when we agonize so much over how we look to others, we fragment this natural unit into two pieces. The result is a continual conflict between our *"appearance body-self"* (how we actually look, how we want the world to see us, how we believe the world sees us) from our *"felt body-self"* (what our body is really telling us about our hunger, our strength, our stamina, our emotional state). When we fragment ourselves in this way we end up feeling disconnected and confused about what's real.

Then, in a bid to fix what we perceive as wrong, we crash diet, or take supplements, or exercise madly. But when we whip our body into shape in this way, without knowing how the human body (and our body in particular) was designed to function best, we not only risk injuring ourselves, we risk forming yet another unnatural armoring in the muscles that serves to control and inhibit rather than support our natural and healthy body responses.

An essential part of being "in shape"—the part most of us forget —is related to our internal fitness, our *joie de vivre,* our relationship to ourselves from the inside out. Once we understand that society's demands on us often go against natural embodiment, we can actively participate in changing our mental/emotional environment to match up with the basic needs of natural health. We can consciously get back into balance.

The first step is to get to know the body we have, to accept it appreciatively, and then ask, What is the best kind of exercise, diet, rest and relaxation, work and play regime for a body such as mine? We would never expect a greyhound to pull a sled or a hippo to run a race against a cheetah. As ludicrous as that sounds, I have met many women who "failed" beginning ballet as children because they were not limber enough or thin enough or their feet and legs couldn't turn out enough. When they got the verdict, they gave up on their bodies altogether. As early as seven or eight years of age, they interpreted their failure at ballet to mean that their bodies were defective. Their minds found their own beautiful bodies guilty of being hopeless klutzes who could never afford to be seen dancing in public again.

The same is true for men. Many men have told me how disempowered they felt because their *stupid bodies* remained scrawny and short throughout high school. They were teased unmercifully by the other boys and even by their fathers and brothers. No matter how well they did in school, having a "hunky" masculine body that excelled in sports was the key to popularity and power. "The girls wouldn't give you a second glance if you weren't on the football, basketball, or soccer team," one still self-conscious man lamented. "Big and strong ruled the school. Even now, as a grown, successful man, I still think size matters most. I'm sure my wife will leave me for a better-looking guy."

That's Not Natural!

We are also subject to societal rules of bodily behavior: Keep your knees together. Don't swing your arms so much. Be still. Don't cry. Don't show your anger, your excitement, your will. These instructions often go against our biology, contradict the natural grace and ease of our movement, and teach us to inhibit our body.

I do not mean to imply that learning to use restraint in certain circumstances is unimportant. Civilized life requires us to learn the difference between bratty behavior, standing up for yourself, and just plain being polite. Our capacity for self-control and discipline is vital to leading a successful and meaningful life. However, these practices are learned best through open education, not through threats and domination. Unfortunately, it is difficult for adults who are already living in bodies they have come to hate to set a good example for children whose pure exuberance can be mistaken for delinquent behavior.

The fact is that when certain physical restraints are continually imposed on the body, our natural posture is forced off balance, sentencing us to a life of unnecessary aches and pains and a general sense of malaise. These inhibitions can become so chronic and habitual that they influence not only our physical posture but our attitudinal stance in the world and toward ourselves. The basis of most of the inhibited body postures you will read about in this section is breathing.

Breathing

Inhale, exhale.

When you're alive, you're breathing. When you're dead, you're not. It would seem to be the simplest, most natural activity in the world. But for many of us, it's not. Unconsciously, we inhale too much and then hold our breath to make up for it, precipitating a panic attack. Or we take tiny little breaths and feel tired from lack of oxygen. Generally, the way we breathe as adults began as a result of our reaction to being told to behave in a way that did not come naturally.

For example, can you remember a time when you were crying and your parent said, "Brave children never cry. Stop that right now!" What did you have to do? How did you adjust your body to stop your tears?

We use our breath and the muscles of the face, throat, chest, upper back, and abdomen to cry. So you probably held your breath while clamping down on your muscles. If you started this practice at three years of age, you're probably pretty good at it by now. In fact, you might not be able to cry now even if you wanted to.

Or perhaps you remember a time when you were so scared you started to cry for help. When no one came, you cried louder and harder and louder and harder until you were hysterical. By the time help arrived, you couldn't stop and it took a long time for you to settle down. Even to this day, when you're up against it you tend to get emotionally out of control.

When we are forced to start inhibiting or exaggerating our expression of sadness, anger, excitement, and happiness at an early age, we run the risk of creating a chronic pattern of muscular holding. Hands-on bodywork techniques such as deep tissue massage combined with natural breathing techniques encourage the body to return to a more natural state of function and response. These methods help release muscle tension, restore a more natural postural alignment with gravity, and reduce stress.

This combination of releasing tension in the muscles with deep breathing can sometimes trigger an emotional release. Especially for people who are chronically tense and withholding, emotional release is an important part of the process of restoring natural balance and tone in the body. It is like the release, refreshment, and cleansing a giant rainstorm brings to a dry meadow. Some people, on the other hand, need to learn how to tolerate and contain their feelings, to learn the difference between the expression and release of natural feeling and hysteria. One way to determine this is to become familiar with the anatomy of breathing, which you can do in the following simple exercise.

Try This Now:

Think of the act of breathing as having four parts.

> **Part 1: Inhale slowly and deeply until your lungs are completely full.**
>
> **Part 2: Notice how you can stay here for a short time if you choose to. I call this "the place of full breath."**
>
> **Part 3: Now, exhale fully until your lungs are completely empty.**
>
> **Part 4: You can also stay in this place for a short time if you want. I call this "the place of no breath."**

We reflect our emotional and mental climates in posture and movement expression, clearly revealing to the educated eye the result of the adversarial relationship between the "natural" body-mind and the "cultural/family" body-mind. Muscle inhibition, combined with poor breathing patterns, can not only reflect but maintain an unnatural body posture fueled by a reactive emotional environment.

Five Unnatural Body Postures: Try Them on for Size!

Let's look now at five basic unnatural body postures. So that you can really experience the way body posture affects breathing, mood, perspective, and emotion, I'm going to ask you to "try them on" as if you were shopping for a new set of body armor (you're not!).

As you read, remember that these postures are *very exaggerated*. We usually express them in far more subtle ways. I have made them cartoon-like to facilitate a sensate experience. When you try each of them on in this over-the-top way, it's easier to feel the substantial consequences of replacing natural posture with an unnatural body armor.

Human beings are complex creatures. As you read, you may identify with more than one of these unnatural postures. Usually, however, you lean toward expressing one version. I hope you enjoy the humor of the process. I'm not making fun of anyone here, but rather getting you acquainted with how neurosis literally takes up

residence in the body so you can learn how important—and possible
—it is to move toward a more natural expression of yourself.

"Poor Me": The Posture of Melancholy

I call people who are suffering from depression or sadness or an
overabundance of melancholy "breath anorexics" because they live
life in the place of no breath. Visualize Eeyore from *Winnie the Pooh*,
or Woody Allen at his most neurotic self, or Charlie Brown from
"Peanuts."

There's a great cartoon that shows Charlie Brown standing lethar-
gically with his head and shoulders bent over, eyes looking down at
the dirt. Lucy cheerfully comes along and says, "Hey Charlie Brown,
wanna play?" He says, "Don't talk to me, I'm depressed." Lucy says
something like, "But Charlie Brown, lift up your head, take a deep
breath and look around. It's a beautiful day, there's not a cloud in the
sky. Let's go play." Without budging, head still down, Charlie Brown
barely lifts his eyes off the ground to look up at Lucy and says, "I
told you, I'm depressed."

The depression that is reflected in the Posture of Melancholy is
fueled by chronic feelings of loss and deprivation. After reaching out
for love, companionship, and acceptance in normal ways, and being
rejected over and over again, these folks fall into a permanent state
of resignation. They recreate their sense of rejection by maintaining
the following stance. Their posture becomes their badge of inferior-
ity and victimization.

Try This Now:

Here's an *exaggerated* example for you to try on. Try this and then
imagine that it feels natural, there are no other options, that this is
you living in your body.

Take in a really deep breath.

**As you exhale every last drop of air out of your lungs
tighten your abdominal muscles, roll your**

shoulders forward, drop your chin to your chest, tighten your jaw, and tuck your pelvis under, like a dog with its tail between its legs.

Now, hold it!

Walk around and notice how you feel.

Now take in a nice big breath, return to normal, and please read on.

Here's how this posture affects the way you relate to the world. First, it shortens the entire front of your body and locks your breath out. Your lung capacity feels smaller, as if you can only swallow a few sips of air at a time. This keeps you feeling tired. In addition, your vision is compromised because your gaze is forced down on the ground in front of you, making you feel that it's an effort just to look where you're going, to notice what's happening in your environment. Your shoulders are frozen to your upper torso. Your arms and hands hang listlessly at your sides, with little capacity to reach out. It's no wonder that so many depressed people report that they have trouble reaching out emotionally. They feel as if no one is there for them—that they are isolated and alone. How ironic that they don't realize the most powerful tools for giving and receiving—their arms—are habitually glued to their sides by a reactive mind combined with an out-of-balance body posture.

Nature did not design the body to look like this. This habitual posture mirrors one's mental reaction to early disappointment, oppression, and defeat.

A melancholy body posture not only reflects a melancholy state of mind, it helps maintain the climate of depression. Learning how to change breathing habits, combined with hands-on bodywork techniques, exercise, and education about the theory of maintaining optimum body responsiveness helps open the chest area and free up natural movement. You feel energized and can literally see what options you have. This process, however, is not magic. The main ingredient required is the will to consciously change. In the comic strip I described, Charlie Brown hadn't made that decision. He was stuck in his feeling of victimization and remained unwilling to see what he might do to change things.

"Me First": The Posture of Emotional Self-Indulgence

I call people who are suffering from hysteria, or too much feeling, emotionally self-indulgent. They live life on an inhalation—most haven't fully exhaled in years. They are gluttons for oxygen, for attention, for fame, fortune, and the good life. Visualize Lucy Ricardo as her most crazed self. She will do anything to get what she wants. Always the adorable clown, she is cunningly out of control. She can seduce anyone but inevitably goes over the top. No matter how silly she gets, though, we always love Lucy. But in real life, emotionally self-indulgent people may not be so lucky, or so lovable. They can get themselves in big trouble with maxed-out credit cards, crowded social calendars, an overabundance of lovers, and chronic exhaustion —with no Ricky to bail them out.

This posture fuels compulsiveness. People who are emotionally self-indulgent have a tendency to spend, spend, spend—to leap before they look—to have big feelings, like thunderstorms that come without warning and blow over quickly. When they're happy, they're *really* happy, when they're angry they're *really* angry, when they're sad, they're *really* sad. They devour life and have a hard time staying grounded. They can be pathologically overbooked, which makes it very difficult to rest within themselves or establish meaningful long-term contact with others.

The hysteria reflected in the Posture of Emotional Self-Indulgence is fueled by a chronic feeling of frustrated desire and the need to be loved. Men and women who have learned that the main ingredient for getting love is to be charming and funny and adorable end up believing that it is far better to look good than to actually feel good. Often spoiled by adoring parents, they fall into a permanent state of giving in order to get. Their posture becomes their badge of specialness, their appearance the only currency they believe they have.

Try This Now:

Here's an *exaggerated* example for you to try on. Try this, and then imagine that it feels natural, that there are no other options, that this is you living in your body. We see this posture more often in women, but men can do it too.

> Quickly take four or five big, deep breaths up into your chest and hold the last one there by locking your diaphragm in place.
>
> Simultaneously, throw your chest out, tuck your tummy in, and arch your pelvis back so that your backside sticks out.
>
> You'll feel like you just drank a strong cappuccino.
>
> You'll look like a helium balloon.
>
> You'll feel as if you have no pelvis or legs—just a huge chest, wanting arms, and bright, active eyes.
>
> You are in a perpetual state of moving toward whatever it is you want in the moment.
>
> Walk around and notice how you feel.
>
> Now exhale, return to normal, and please read on.

This posture lengthens and expands the entire front of your body while shortening the back and pulling the lower spine into a lordotic (or swaybacked) curve. It locks your breath in. Your lung capacity will feel huge, like you can swallow a whole lot of air at once. This keeps you highly energized (sometimes to the point of feeling giddy) and on the go, go, go. Your eyes glitter above a buoyant chest that keeps you looking out into the world for the things you want. Your arms and hands reach out with little awareness of what is behind you. You are all front with no back—all arms, chest, and eyes, with no legs. Your mind, when it thinks, imagines you are having fun, but your disregarded body often doesn't agree. You exist primarily from the waist up, keeping those pesky genitals held back by the outward curve of the lower spine.

Nature did not design the body to look like this. This habitual posture mirrors an early emotional/mental reaction to frustrated desire, and to the fear of disapproval.

It's no wonder so many emotionally self-indulgent people report they have trouble relaxing. They feel as if they can't get off the merry-go-round of life, but they can't bear to be alone. How ironic that they don't even realize the most powerful tools for feeling grounded, calm, and relaxed—their pelvis, legs, and feet—are habitually abandoned by their out-of-balance body posture.

"I'm the Boss": The Posture of Aggression

I call people who wield a chronic attitude of aggression that says "I'm the boss here, don't mess with me" Alpha Dogs. Like the emotionally self-indulgent types, these people live life on an inhalation, but with a different pattern of muscle tension. They use the muscles of the face, chest, back, and spine like a shield of armor that allows them to breathe in a way that reveals nothing about themselves. They subscribe to a survival-of-the-fittest philosophy and are incessantly ready to save the day or get their way. Visualize John Wayne walking into a bar filled with bad guys, or Clint Eastwood challenging an adversary with the words "Make my day."

This person will do anything to get what he (or she) wants—the girl or the guy, the bad guys, the power. Aggressive types are always on guard, admirably defiant, and completely in control—mentally, emotionally, and physically.

They know how to dominate anyone, but at what price? In the movies, the good guy Alpha Dogs always win the war and get the girl, while the bad guy Alpha Dogs don't. In real life, most Alpha Dogs are destined to remain emotionally unavailable and locked up in their bodies, leaving little capacity for empathy and joy, which usually means failing miserably at intimate relationships.

This posture fuels anger and isolation. Alpha Dogs live hard. They tend to alienate their loved ones with out-of-control rage and accusation, making them feel unloved and locked out because they have such a hard time expressing emotion and feeling sensation.

The aggression in this posture is fueled by a chronic need to feel powerful and in control. These folks learned early on that the way to feel powerful was to be intimidating, unemotional, and cunning. Often disciplined by an Alpha Dog parent, these people fall into a permanent state of defending the realm. Their posture becomes their badge of courage. Perhaps more than any other posture type, Alpha Dogs demand respect by maintaining the following stance.

Try This Now:

Here's an *exaggerated* example of the posture of aggression for you to try on. Try this and then imagine that it feels natural, that you have no other options, that this is you living in your body. We see this posture more often in men, but women can do it too.

> Stand with your feet a bit wider than shoulder distance apart.
>
> Take in a long, deep breath.
>
> As you do, tighten your buttocks muscles and pull your chin into your chest while keeping your face front, your eyes on the horizon line.
>
> Now hold it.
>
> Hold your arms and hands vigilantly at your sides, ready to draw your guns.
>
> When you want to see something, you have to turn your whole body because your neck is glued to your torso, your torso is glued to your waist, your waist is glued to your pelvis. Your torso is one solid, unbending mass.
>
> Someone could punch you in the stomach and you wouldn't feel a thing.
>
> You could punch someone else in the stomach and not feel a thing.
>
> And that's the intention of this armoring stance: not to feel a thing.

No pain. No pleasure. No remorse. No joint mobility.

Just lots of power and invulnerability.

It is a hero's stance at best.

A bully's stance at worst.

Walk around and notice how you feel.

Now exhale, inhale, return to normal, and please
read on.

This defensive posture strengthens and hardens the muscles of
the entire front of the body, not to mention the back and the deep
internal muscles. When the muscles of the chest in particular are
immobilized, anger and sexual desire are about the only feelings that
register. You feel huge, powerful, dense, and in charge. Your eyes are
frozen and unfeeling above an iron body that keeps them looking out
into the world for dangerous adventure. Your arms and hands are
ready for conflict. You are mostly back with little front—a rigid spine
and pelvis with no legs to support you. Visualize a male body builder,
a huge inflated torso on top of thin spindly legs on the bottom. You
treat your body like a junkyard dog and haven't had a feeling in years.

Nature did not design the body to look like this. This habitual
posture mirrors an early physical/emotional reaction to the fear of
showing weakness. Softening the muscles of the chest and opening
the joints of the entire body, combined with permission to exhale, can
make the world come alive with color and meaning. It might even
lower blood pressure or make a grown man cry.

"Going and Going and Going": The Posture of the Overachiever

I call people who suffer from an overabundance of ambitious
energy Overachievers. Overachievers live life in the middle of an inhalation. They breathe in just enough, lock their diaphragm in neu-
tral, and then go, go, go. Visualize the Energizer Bunny or the typical
Type A personality.

The attitude reflected in the posture of the overachiever is fueled
by an obsessive need to win, an unbending notion that failure is

taboo. From childhood, Overachievers play the game of exchanging victory for love. If you lost the race or got a B instead of an A or acted weird, you didn't exist. These folks are in a permanent state of doing. Their posture becomes their badge of excellence. They recreate their sense of living to win by maintaining the following stance.

Try This Now:

Here's an *exaggerated* example for you to try on. Try this and then imagine that it feels natural, that there are no other options, that this is you living in your body.

> Grab onto something in the distance with your eyes.
>
> Stare at it hard.
>
> Don't let it out of your sight.
>
> You've got to have it.
>
> You've got to get there, no matter what.
>
> Your eyes bear down.
>
> Your eyes are all you need to get ahead.
>
> Your vision narrows.
>
> Your head juts out as far ahead of your body as possible.
>
> You cut off all contact between your head and your body.
>
> Your breath is neither deep nor shallow.
>
> You are all front with no back.
>
> You go toward the desired object or plan like a bull with blinders on.
>
> Anyone who gets in your way will have your footprints on their back.
>
> You must be the winner.
>
> Nothing else matters.
>
> Not your health.

Not your friends.

Not your environment.

This is the posture of Silicon Valley, where the hard
   drive reigns—where tomorrow cancels out
   yesterday—where success rules.

Walk around and notice how you feel.

Now breathe deeply, return to normal, and please
   read on.

This is the typical Type A body posture. It is perfect for maintaining high blood pressure. It can lead to eventual collapse from
chronic fatigue whether you are physically fit or out of shape. That's
because there is no internal world hook-up here—there is little respect for the natural limitations of bodily life. Getting the job done
requires complete attention to work—to the outside world's competitive marketplace. Relaxation is not easily cultivated by Overachievers. It might even feel threatening.

This posture deadens the body. When the muscles are anesthe-
tized it is easier to push forward, no matter what—to have no doubt
that you will win. Overachievers look out toward the winner's circle
with bright and unfeeling eyes from a head that is always ahead of
the game. Whether that head is perched above a well-oiled Mercedes
Benz of a body or a real clunker makes no difference. In either case,
arms and hands are held ready to exploit.

These Overachievers are all about image. It's as if they couldn't
find the time to learn how to use the spine, pelvis, and legs for
support—for the actual feeling of integrity. Visualize Bill Gates or
Rupert Murdoch or Madonna. The motto is: Push your body to the
max. Resting is for wimps. I can smell the roses in my hotel room
while I'm changing clothes. Overachievers are more than willing to
work eight days a week and have little sympathy for those who can't
take the heat.

Nature did not design the body to look like this. This habitual
posture mirrors an emotional/physical reaction to the unbearable fear
of failure. A deep tissue massage designed to soften muscles and open
the joints of the entire body through breath and touch can make the

world slow down and come alive with sensation and meaning for the Overachiever. It might even make a grownup want to stay and watch the sunset.

"Don't Rock the Boat": The Posture of Compliance

I call people who suffer from an underabundance of ambitious energy Over-Compliant. Over-Compliants live life in the place of easy breath, they don't sigh and they don't gulp. They breathe in just enough, relax to the point of sloppiness, and then hang out. Visualize R. Crumb's "Keep on Truckin'" cartoon character, Mr. Natural; or Gilligan from *Gilligan's Island;* or the classic surfer dude or vacant-faced hippie—"Whatever's right, man."

The attitude reflected in the Posture of Compliance is fueled by an obsessive need to not make waves, to avoid conflict, and an unbending notion that winning is taboo. From childhood, Compliants played the game of exchanging agreeable behavior for love. If you stayed cool, if you didn't need anything, you were valuable. Making a scene was the best way to lose. These folks might claim they are at peace, but actually they are in a perpetual state of waiting. Their posture is their cover. They recreate their sense of living to comply by maintaining the following stance.

Try This Now:

Here's an *exaggerated* example for you to try on. Try this and then imagine it feels natural, that there are no other options, that this is you living in your body.

> Imagine you are a rag doll, or maybe a sloth.
>
> Your eyes are unfocused, your attention diffuse.
>
> The word hurry does not exist in your vocabulary.
>
> Don't focus on anything.
>
> That way you don't have to want, or help, or participate with life.

You don't have to have anything, and you don't need
   to get anywhere.

Your head rests atop a torso that slouches lazily,

that leans back and expects your legs to carry it, to do
   all the work.

That's how you cut off contact between thinking and
   feelings.

Your breathing is lazy.

You are "laid back, man," claiming little attachment to
   fashion and formality.

You are an expert at waiting.

You go "with" rather than "toward" or "against" the
   desired plan.

You get along with everyone and initiate next to
   nothing.

You must feel comfortable.

Nothing else matters.

Not your health.

Not your friends.

Not your feelings.

This is the posture of the "Surfer Dude," where time
   is irrelevant and computers superfluous—where
   peace and love win over success and power—
   where right now is all there is—where going with
   the flow is the only option.

Walk around and notice how you feel.

Now breathe deeply, return to normal,
   and please read on.

This is *way* past the typical Type B body posture. It is perfect for
maintaining a low-key lifestyle and underachievement. It is often supported by functional alcohol abuse and wasted talents. These folks

have little respect for the intelligence of the mind and scant desire to know how to know. They mistake their passivity for peacefulness and end up missing out on much of what life has to offer. They don't want to know who they really are or what they really want. Conscious awareness is not easily cultivated by Compliants. It's too much trouble.

This posture deadens the mind and the heart, but in quite a different way than the Overachiever Type A posture. This is a mindless deadening that often leads to a life of pure physicality, such as round-the-clock skiing or sailing or surfing. When our brain is lazy, it is easier to forget what we want—to have any desire to go forward to see what's on the other side of the mountain. Compliants look out with half-opened sleepy eyes perched above an unkempt, friendly body. Arms and hands hang lazily at the sides but are quite alive, well used, and coordinated. Lifting the spine is just too much work. Visualize Pooh Bear with his honey jar in tow. The motto is: Don't rock the boat. Take it easy. Don't worry, be happy.

But nature did not design the body to look like this either. As calm as it is, this posture is a reaction formation to being overlooked in childhood, to learning early on it doesn't pay to drive in the fast lane. Breath work combined with joint manipulation designed to open the muscles to sensation and release pent-up emotions can energize the mind and wake these sleepy people up. It might even make them want to think more deeply about where they're going as they sail through life.

The Posture of Natural Design

Dr. Moshe Feldenkrais, innovator of the Awareness Through Movement system, said, "Learning that is not conducted through a new way of action is not learning. Learning is a crystallization of experience." How would we move if the body were left to its own intelligence and allowed to develop in a natural way? This is almost impossible to conceive of in a culture like ours that encourages all sorts of body shaping and exercise regimens, and from early childhood on asks us to sit still in uncomfortable chairs and be quiet!

The body was not made for regular repetitive exercise, like typing at your computer for eight hours at a clip, or jogging for miles, day in and day out. Problems such as carpal tunnel syndrome and tendonitis are usually the result of such mind-driven effort.

Left to its own intelligence, the body would never run so many miles a day on pavement, or do strenuous workouts on a Stairmaster day after day after day, or run for miles on a treadmill at the gym while staring at the wall. (Did you know that treadmills got their start as a way for prisoners to work off energy?) This kind of exercise often does more harm than good because your body is not in alignment to begin with. Your legs can't stay strong and healthy when your knees are knocking or your ankles are weakened by feet that roll in.

Left to its own intelligence, the body regulates itself by listening for the actual sensations of needs such as hunger, fear, anger, interest, exhaustion, sexual arousal, pleasure, and joy. No animal in nature runs for miles on an asphalt surface just to stay in shape. When animals run for fun they stop and start, sprint and trot, leap and change directions. When they run for their lives, that's another story. Nature in its wisdom designed us very well. Too bad we took it upon our neurotic minds to redesign our user manuals.

Think about it from the body's point of view. The force of gravity holds us to the earth. When the body is out of alignment, gravity can't be evenly distributed. For example, when your head is chronically thrust forward, the force of gravity hits you where your cervical spine sticks out beyond the rest of your torso. Eventually, your neck will begin to hurt.

Try This Now:

Take a moment to reconnect with your body as it is right now. Don't judge it, just notice it.

> Walk around the room just the way you always do.
>
> Don't change anything.
>
> What does it feel like to live in your body right now?
>
> Are your feet turned out, turned in, or pointed straight ahead?
>
> Is your stride short or long?

Does your weight come down harder on your right or left foot?

On the heel or ball of your foot?

Does one arm swing more easily from the shoulder than the other?

Where is your vision focused:

On the ground, the horizon, or darting all around?

Are you breathing fully?

Is your chest expanding or contracted?

Is your jaw loose or tight?

Is your tongue relaxed, or pressed against the inside of your mouth?

Is your lower back arched out or tucked under?

Do you feel pain or discomfort anywhere in your body?

Now Try This:

Try changing your posture to see how it feels.

Try walking with your feet turned way out like a duck, then way in like a pigeon.

Walk with all your weight on the outside of your foot, then on the inside.

Notice how the position of your feet affects your body all the way up to your neck.

Most of us do a less exaggerated version of one of the above walks. Your body is designed to work best with your feet pointing straight ahead, with your weight coming down evenly through the center of your feet, with your ankles and knees lined up evenly under your hips.

The act of walking begins with bending the knee. This allows the leg to lift up and swing forward like an arm. When you balance on the supporting leg as the moving leg swings through, you can naturally place your foot onto the floor. This is different from throwing your body weight onto the swinging leg as if you were preventing a fall. When you do this, the knee and hip get a lot more wear and tear. When you do this with your feet turned out or in, your knees get twisted in ways they weren't designed to work.

Try Walking Like This Instead:

Feel how the vertebrae of your spine are like a string of beads rather than a steel rod.

Imagine that you are lifted up effortlessly by an invisible string attached to a point on the back of the top of your skull.

At the same time, feel how gravity is radiating down through your bones and muscles—your feet firmly planted on the ground.

You are heavy and light at the same time.

Feel the spaciousness in your spine.

Feel the lightness in your pelvis that makes it easier to swing the legs from your hips and relax your lower back while standing still or walking.

Breathe deeply.

Allow your head to float on your neck, your eyes to relax so your peripheral vision can tell you more about where you are, your jaw to loosen, your tongue to relax.

Feel your back.

Feel yourself in the space around you.

Feel that your body is a container for yourself.

Feel that your body is multidimensional: it has a top,
    a bottom, sides, a back, and a front.

Feel how you are connected to the earth.

Now you can reach for the sky.

This is not your mother talking.

This is not charm school protocol.

It is the voice of your natural body intelligence.

CHAPTER 4

Telling Your Story from the Voice of Your Body

In order to break out of a prison, one must first confess to being in a prison

— WILHELM REICH

After so many years of living with muscle armor that shuts down or obscures the message of your instincts and senses, you will have to make an initial effort to listen to your body intelligence. Living with senses wide open begins by being willing to consciously interrupt your old artificial habits of mind, heart, and body and replace them with the ways nature designed you to function. I don't want to mislead you: It takes a degree of discipline, study, and passion to commit to practicing natural embodiment combined with awareness.

First things first. Just as you clean a cup before pouring in fresh water, you need to clear out the old story you've been telling yourself about how life works before a fresh, more honest vision can take root. You must be willing to see how you are out of balance before you can consciously change. Listen to Janice's story—it's an example of how much influence body-centered education can have, even when our initial resistance is great.

Janice's Story: No Pain No Gain

Janice is a fiercely driven, work-obsessed Silicon Valley marketing executive. At age thirty-seven, she was hardly living. Her serious approach to everything, including vacations, kept her inflexible and humorless.

When Janice enrolled in a class I was teaching, she said it was because she wanted to learn the skill of hands-on bodywork as a second job opportunity. I've always suspected her unconscious drove her to finally explore this other side of the tracks—a world that values body and soul more than success and prestige.

The going was rough in the beginning. Despite my passionate lectures and demonstrations on the importance of learning how to touch another person with sensitivity and kindness, with unconditional regard, Janice just didn't get it. She related to the bodies of her classmates as if they were machines that needed to be fixed. Her touch was mechanical, rigid, and demanding. Her inability to recognize this made it impossible for me to graduate her so she could move on to more advanced training. Accustomed to excelling at everything, Janice was outraged. She was sure I was incorrectly evaluating her work. I recommended that we do a few one-on-one sessions to see if we could work things out.

Janice began our first session by complaining about how uncomfortable the chair was and asking me to close the window and dim the overhead light. When I asked her what else was wrong in her life, out poured a litany of complaints. From her perspective, nobody could get it right. She had a hard time sleeping because the neighbors were too noisy. She hated driving because everyone broke the speed limit. She hated shopping because she could never find clothes that fit her properly, and on and on and on.

Curiously, her irritation was triggered by imperfections in the physical world around her. Not only did she suffer from pain in her body in general, but her senses were geared to smelling out what stank. Janice hardly ever noticed the fragrance of a rose or the sound of leaves rustling on a summer's day. She used her senses to justify her discontent.

I pointed this out to Janice and asked her what she made of my observation. With a puzzled look, she shrugged her shoulders and said, "So, what does that have to do with anything? There's a lot in life that stinks."

It was apparent to me that Janice's body was so rigid and controlled—so shut off from pleasure—that she would have trouble comprehending the notion that the body has a voice. In fact, she did not hesitate to say she thought it was a silly, irrational idea. "My body can't think, let alone talk," she said emphatically.

I asked her what she thought the purpose of pain and pleasure were, of grief and joy, of fear and comfort? She said, "Sensations and feelings are things to control and conquer. Otherwise they get in the way of progress." So it made perfect sense when she finally told me the story of what happened to her body as she was growing up, that her reality was controlled by the voice of her earnestly judgmental mind. It was going to take some time for Janice to learn how to speak from the voice of her body.

Maintaining her stiff, upright posture as she sat in the chair before me, Janice said she could not recall ever being held by either her mother or her father. As she dutifully described her family life, I could see her irritation growing as she tightened her lips over her teeth and clenched her jaw. Without knowing it, she was showing me how she had learned to bite back her anger and swallow it down into her belly where it festered into resentment and blame. It was painful to witness.

Clearly Janice did not like talking about her childhood. She looked for a way to change the subject. She would rather complain about the inadequacies she saw all around her—about the pain and discomfort she presently felt in her own overworked body, about the life we are given in general. She was critical of just about everything, and had little sympathy for anyone. I expected her to write a letter to God about what a bad job he'd done with the Earth.

Nevertheless, I tried to stay the course, and urged her to continue telling me about her family. Passionlessly, Janice reported that her family life had been very disciplined and emotionally constrained. Her parents had no hugs for her, and they didn't touch each other either. Janice was the black sheep of the family. She was sent to boarding school starting at age eleven. There she was taught to value high academic achievement and a tireless work ethic above all else. She lived in a world of mind over matter and didn't even know it.

Janice's body had become the enemy. Her mother had regularly told her how to hide her "unattractive features," and from early on Janice had judged herself skinny, awkward, and ugly.

"I was very shy," she said. "I was sure that the other kids didn't want to play with me, so I played alone. I have always felt very alone."

Her tone was bitter, and she did not look at me as she continued on with her story. "In boarding school and college it was the same. I have suffered from bad headaches and a general feeling of stiffness throughout my body as long as I can remember."

I pointed out to Janice that it seemed to me the only way she had found to survive her childhood was to shut off her positive feelings and good sensations, replacing them with judgments, rules, and strong ambition. To add insult to injury, she was continuing to do so as an adult. She hated the dish life had served her. Her negativity only made her irritable and persnickety. Her anger fueled her arduous workout schedule. Nothing could make her *not* jog those seven miles a day and then work out with weights at her local gym. "No pain, no gain" was definitely her motto. It was time for me to reiterate my theories about the connection between pleasure and health.

I gave her some books to read about human behavior. I wanted to feed her mind, to get her thinking in new ways about the dilemma of being human. Janice was astonished to learn her responses were fairly predictable—that there was an explanation for her duty-driven, pleasureless life that went beyond her childhood experiences. She seemed relieved to hear that research had identified different types of body armor that supported different types of ego structures. (Janice was a complicated combination of the Posture of Depression and the Posture of the Overachiever, with a touch of the Posture of Aggression.)

The somatic approach could provide a map of her conditioned tendency and how to change it. Janice was not a one-of-a-kind freak of nature, as she had so often feared. There were others very much like her, people who treated their bodies like machines, people who were overly self-disciplined with unreasonably high expectations of themselves and the others in their lives. Their bodies, like hers, were often rigid and closed off to feelings and sensations.

This realization, combined with ongoing bodywork and movement awareness classes, enabled Janice to understand physically as well as intellectually that her painful body rigidity was the armor she used to keep her emotions and desires locked away inside her. It would take some more time for her to soften, for her to see herself with more compassion and acceptance, but she was off to a good start.

Write Your Autobiography from the Voice of Your Body

Like Janice, most of us regulate our behavior out of reaction to a convincing cognitive mistake made in childhood. If you can remember how, why, and when you were forced to contain or distort bodily expressions like joy, fear, anger, and sadness, you can evaluate these choices in the present and clear the way for change. If you can remember a time when you were completely un-self-conscious in your own body, when you were bathing in your senses with no critical self-witness torturing you to do something useful, you can begin to cultivate that state once again.

As you write your story, allow yourself to flow, to put down whatever comes up. Please don't get hung up on producing perfect prose. We don't have much practice or permission in our culture to describe the various hues of sensation. Just take a moment, feel your body, and let it speak from pen to paper in incomplete phrases. Your mind will understand later when you read over what you have written.

If you don't feel comfortable writing a story, just begin with a simple list. Here's an example:

Age 3:

I loved pretending to be a frog. Mom delighted in my leaping and all was right with the world.

Age 5:

I fell off a stool in the bathroom, cracked my head open, and had to get stitches. They tied me down in the emergency room and yelled at me for screaming.

Age 6:

I got beat up at school and was afraid to go back, but I did anyway. Dad said to fight back next time, so I did. I beat the shit out of Danny Miller and felt powerful. I decided to be the bully from then on.

Age 7:

My favorite thing was playing with my dog. We got real dirty and I loved to eat dog cookies.

Age 8:

Mom took me to ballet class. I was the only one whose feet wouldn't turn out all the way. I hated it. I've felt like a klutz ever since.

What can you do with this story? Your muscles remember. By evoking memory you evoke feeling and sensation in spite of your story line. If you can let yourself remember or reexperience the actual feeling of childhood joy and freedom, you can jump-start it now. Likewise, once you realize how a terrifying childhood trauma locked fear and repression into your body, you can begin to reeducate yourself and let the fear go.

Or, you could tell a memory like this:

I remember when I was five years old. I took off all my clothes and was dancing around the backyard smelling the fresh grass, feeling the warm sun on my little face and naked body when Dad ran out and yelled at me. "What do you think you're doing young lady? Put your clothes back on and go to your room. I am so ashamed of you!" Ever since I have not only been overly modest, but very shy about dancing and being seen in general.

What can you do with this story? If your adult self sees how both you and your father overreacted, and now you don't believe it is shameful for a five-year-old to dance around naked, you can begin to practice allowing your body to move more freely.

The experience of how you have held your breath and tightened your muscles for years so as not to feel too exuberant causes you to begin breathing deeply now. Your new awareness cheers you on because you know that this is a most important ingredient for feeling connected—for enjoying your life.

This process will help stimulate your ability to distinguish the difference between thoughts in the mind and sensations in the body. It is a primary step in the process of reclaiming three-dimensional living—of allowing the actual experience of pleasure to be an active part of your life.

Try This Now:

> Put this book down and get out your journal or a
> small notebook.
>
> You are going to begin to write your autobiography
> from the voice of your body.
>
> That means remembering the smells, tastes, sounds,
> sensations, colors, and images that seasoned your
> life's experiences and colored your thoughts.
>
> Breathe deeply as you remember how you have
> learned to live.
>
> Now, tell your own story.

Learn From Your Story

With your story in front of you, you can begin to learn how the body's messages are reflected in the body's muscle tensions, habitual posture, habits of touch, voice tone, and knee-jerk responses. No matter how good we are at separating mind and body, each inevitably affects the other. The first step toward understanding the connection between mind and body is to understand the difference between your romanticized story ("My childhood? It was fine. My parents stayed together, unlike most of my friends' families.") and what actually happened ("My Dad was at work most of the time, my Mom took care of us. Mom and Dad never argued, but they didn't talk much either.")

Remembering the events that caused your body to build its emotional and physical defenses (tense and inhibiting or flaccid and unresponsive muscle armor, oversensitivity or undersensitivity, taking in and holding your breath or never quite getting enough breath) is an essential part of learning how to let go. Remembering the moments that brought you joy and allowed your body to act freely is also essential for learning how to reunite with the natural intelligence that is your birthright.

Telling your story in the presence of a trustworthy witness such as a body-oriented psychotherapist or educator can help to illuminate how some of your memories still have the power to evoke the same emotional expression and the same body armoring that they did when you were younger. Now you're a grownup. You know what your rights are and have the authority to use your mind and senses to see reality more accurately, protect yourself and take your power back. Once you are able to see how frightening and painful memories have the power to keep you stuck in a reactive trap—how you have become so habituated to your own methods of repression that you fail to recognize them as defense mechanisms—you can seek an unbiased witness to mentor you in the process of seeing yourself more clearly, someone who can teach you how to develop the focus and courage to actually change, to take charge of your own life.

When you add a movement discipline such as yoga or t'ai chi to your practice, or start to get some bodywork, you will learn how to recognize and even interrupt the old worn-out habits that grab onto your body, heart, and mind. Telling your autobiography from the voice of your body prepares you for the next step in the process of choosing to live consciously in your body: practicing a body-centered discipline.

Practice Body-Centered Awareness

Our society rewards us for *thinking* our way in and out of situations. It's no wonder so many people feel they are "leading with their heads," as if they will topple over at any moment. The closer we get to living harmoniously with mind, heart, and body, the less disjointed and off balance we feel. More and more, as we feel the ground firmly under our feet, we move from our center.

So it makes sense that the next step is actually to practice body awareness. That means regularly taking the time to notice the difference between sensation and thought, and then learning how to encourage your body to be more naturally responsive, flexible, and strong. Regular practice—such as yoga, t'ai chi, martial arts, and movement awareness classes—teach you how to make contact with the body's intelligence.

Even if you can't take classes, you can still practice on your own. For example, feeling the sensation of the weight of gravity as it bears down through your bones and muscles leads you to naturally adjust yourself when you get out of balance. When you take your cues from actual body-centered feedback, you understand why respecting the body's signals is essential to an overall sense of ease. Operating from the philosophy that you *are* your body—that body intelligence is key to your success as a humane and healthy being—makes it imperative to refuse the cultural call to whip the body into shape. As long as you feel like your body is a stranger who just came along for the ride, you will find it difficult to relax into it or trust your instinctive responses.

Practice Breathing

In addition to developing an active body-centered discipline, simple breath techniques combined with hands-on bodywork, such as regular deep tissue massage, can also help awaken the ability to distinguish between "good" pain and "bad" pain; between tension and hypersensitivity; between thoughts in the mind, sensations in the body, and emotional expression.

Attending to the sensation of breath as you inhale through your nose is a cornerstone of simple meditation. Meditation is a way to find your center; it provides the mind with a stabilized focus of attention that helps to stop habitual mental chit-chat. This is how you learn to pay attention to what actually *is* rather than to what your out-of-control thought process thinks should or shouldn't be.

As long as you are alive, you breathe. Because energy follows attention, you tend to vary your breathing pattern unconsciously according to what you are doing. When you are concentrating on solving a difficult math problem, for example, you may hold your breath. When you are anxious about someone you love making it home safely in a driving snowstorm, you may take many shallow breaths.

By learning to focus on the sensation of breath as you inhale, you can successfully interrupt your preoccupation with thinking, with trying to rewrite your life (for a little while, at least). The conscious act of suspending the thinking process stimulates the ability to see life as it really is. This allows you to respond more honestly and appropriately, to be more fully present.

Try This Now:

> Turn off everything: the phone, the TV, the computer.
>
> Sit in a comfortable chair or on a pillow on the floor.
>
> Cross your legs and keep your spine straight, your body alert and relaxed at the same time.
>
> Now close your eyes.
>
> Place your attention on the sensation of breath as you inhale through your nose.
>
> When your mind wanders, gently bring it back to the sensation of breath, period.
>
> Do this for ten minutes.
>
> When you are finished, take out your journal and write about what you noticed.

Janice's Story Continued: Stress Reduction Equals Pleasure Induction

Now that you've given yourself and your own story some time and thought, let's go back to Janice. Inspired by what she was learning and how she was changing, Janice entered into the serious study of body-mind philosophy and psychology. Still, she remained suspicious of my claim that the need for pleasure was inherent. I asked her to try something very simple: taking a hot bath, but with complete awareness and attention.

Janice, true to form, reacted to the very idea. "Take a hot bath!" she smirked. "Come on, this is getting too New Age-y for me to take seriously."

"Trust me." I said. "Just give it a try. If you don't like it, you can tell me and that will lead us somewhere else."

I recommend you try it too, when you have some time.

Try This in the Privacy of Your Own Home:

You are going to take a hot bath. Make sure you can be alone for at least one hour.

Before you begin, unplug the phones—all of them—your cellular phone, your pager. Turn off the TV and radio.

Prepare the bathroom as if you were drawing a bath for your beloved. Clean the tub.

Put out clean towels and a robe. Choose a soap, bath salts if you like, and candles with a fragrance you love.

Before you step in the tub, run the water and make sure the room is warm enough. Have a glass of fresh water or juice in easy reach. Now you are ready to start the exercise.

> Take a moment to shift your attention from thinking to sensation.
>
> Let your mind go and open your senses.
>
> This is a meditation practice.
>
> Take off your clothes slowly, noticing every sensation.
>
> What is it like to stand naked, without judgment?
>
> With what part of your body do you test the water to see if it is hot enough?
>
> How do you lower yourself into the tub?
>
> And so it goes.
>
> Keep bringing your attention back to sensation.
>
> Breathe deeply as you bathe in the realm of your senses.
>
> Take your time. There is no place else to go.
>
> Let your body tell you what it wants.

If the water gets too cold, run some hot water.

If you are thirsty, drink.

If you want to change position, change.

If you want to move in the water, move.

When your mind tells you that you're wasting time, stay in the tub.

When your body wants to get out of the tub, get out.

Notice the sensation of emerging from hot water, of being wet in the dry air, of the towel on your skin, of the texture of the floor beneath your bare feet.

Once you are out and dry, lie down on your bed for a while, or stretch, or listen to your favorite music.

Allow your psyche to absorb this experience, to store it in your body's memory bank.

This is essential. Enjoy the moment.

Janice's Bath Experience

Janice came to our next appointment with a more relaxed look on her face and a million observations. "I had the best night's sleep I've had in years after I took my bath," she said. "The bath itself was difficult. My mind wanted to evaluate everything. It was all I could do to feel even the heat of the water. I could hear your voice asking me to bring my attention back to sensation, but then my mind would take over and I'd be unhappy with my choice of soap. I'd tell myself, 'You should have chosen the jasmine,' stupid things like that. But I did it, and I see that there is something to this focusing-on-sensation business. The bath really did relax me. I think I even felt better the whole next day."

Janice Opens Up

It took a year of classes and sessions, practice and respectful self-discipline for Janice to really bring the language of the body into her life. She was beginning to understand the essential role natural embodiment and pleasure play in the process of relieving stress and enhancing contact. She was willing to be easier on herself during her workouts, to take more time off, to set better boundaries around her work schedule in general.

Janice was starting to look relaxed and open. She reported how amazed she was by how much pleasure and serenity she was able to feel, at how much better she was sleeping through the night. She had no idea of what her body was capable of, at how deprived she had kept herself.

Everything began to open up once Janice allowed herself to respond to the phenomenal pleasures of the body in balance—to see that the act of generously receiving what is given is key to the feeling of joy. She began to come to our sessions with tales of her new-found tolerance, patience, and downright generosity of spirit at work and with her family. She actually began to enjoy her colleagues instead of seeing them as sources of problems that needed fixing. She even looked wonderful, her beauty clearly emanating from the inside out. She took vacations for the first time, and began to value and enjoy her private time alone. Even though her old habits still raised their ugly heads from time to time, and probably would for the rest of her life, Janice knew she was actively engaged with her life, she knew how to bring herself back to center. In response, her bodywork was becoming kind and effective, her own body felt far less achy and rigid, and she was much easier to get to know. Janice had finally come home to her body.

Keep a Body Journal

As you begin to explore your body history, it is important to be gentle with yourself and brutally honest at the same time. You must be willing to accept the fact that you—along with every other person in the world—have gone through life continually putting your own biased spin on whatever happens. Life changes when you are willing to see things the way they are as opposed to the way you want them to be. Your senses are an important ally in learning to choose the present over the past.

Try This Now:

> **Keep a body-story journal for a week and see how your awareness changes.**

For example:

Monday:
On the way to work today I started to have an anxiety attack. I thought I was going to be late. My mouth got dry and my heart started pounding as I began to worry about what the boss would say. As it turned out, I made it to work on time but I felt out of sorts all day and didn't get much accomplished.

Tuesday:
Every time I started to worry about being late on the way to work, I shifted my attention to my breath. I put on my favorite CD and willed myself to hear without naming. It really worked. Before I knew it, my body relaxed and I was able to lean back and enjoy the ride. I kept telling my worried self, "There's nothing you can do. Worrying will not get you there any sooner. So open your senses and take this time to relax while remaining alert rather than hyper and paranoid." When I got to work I noticed that I was able to stay in a good mood all day. I didn't get my usual four o'clock headache.

What's in It for You?

Well, I've asked you to do quite a few things in one short chapter: tell the story of your life, take a hot bath, and keep track of your daily body sensations. At this point you may be wondering if the commitment to body-centered awareness is worth all the effort of changing patterns you've grown used to over the years.

It is.

When we lose trust in the body's instinctive responses, we end up like Sarah, in Chapter One. Because she didn't understand that instinctive fear works from a reflex that happens automatically when we are in real danger, she couldn't see how she was creating unnecessary stress by thinking fearful thoughts. We need the feeling of fear to release adrenaline so we can fight or run. But when fear is a constant mental concern, we lose all sense of balance. Thinking becomes paranoid and ineffectual. The body becomes a slave to the false alarms set off by a fearful mind. Stress builds and builds, making relaxation almost impossible. In other words, this sense of center is not just physical: It has a mental component too.

We preserve a sense of center by sustaining the qualities of clarity, impartiality, and acceptance—mentally, physically, and emotionally. A strong sense of center helps us determine the difference between imagination and reality.

An increased sensate awareness also teaches us about the true nature of our instincts. As we learn to stop looking through a past-memory filter and perceive what we are feeling right now—through the continual input of sight, sound, touch, taste, and smell—we learn to respond to people and life situations more appropriately. We become less inhibited and more ourselves.

This is fundamental to building intimate healthy relationships with others and with the world around us. The bonding response, for example, is a natural outcome of loving-kindness—as instinctive as the fight/flight response. It is stimulated and sustained by the direct experience of pleasure and is transmitted through such relationships as parenting, friendship, and sexuality. When we learn to respond naturally, using all of our senses and allowing the conscious mind to work with the innate intelligence of the body, we naturally increase our capacity for empathy and naturally expand our sense of connection to the world. This ability to enter into the feeling or spirit of another person, place, or thing is a primary ingredient of healthy relating.

CHAPTER 5

Touch: The Pattern That Connects

Not only our geometry and our physics, but our whole conception of what exists outside us, is based on the sense of touch.

—BERTRAND RUSSELL

Recently, I was visiting some dear friends and their bright-eyed one-year-old son. One morning, they invited me into their bedroom to use the telephone. I found them naked together in their big comfy king-sized bed. They were definitely a sensate unit. The baby treated his parents' bodies, especially his mom's, like they belonged to him. He was still nursing, and her breasts were his territory. He romped and played, diving beneath the soft down comforter to play peek-a-boo one minute, and jumping up and down on the mattress the next. Mom and Dad were laughing, making goofy noises, faces and gestures. They were all delightfully comfortable together.

I felt warmed, aroused in a pleasant sort of way. How amazing it was to feel the raw sensuality that was present in this family. Even though I knew that I could not enter into this sacred alliance, I recognized my own deep longing for this same kind of union. I couldn't help but ask myself, is this what we all really want from one another? Is this the feeling of deep intimacy, the lost voice of the instinctive body calling for a return to the unselfconscious expression of delight?

Our culture has come to see sexuality as something separate from regular life. Sex has become that dirty dance we do with our genitals

—that disconnected but powerful part of ourselves we often can't control and certainly don't feel comfortable about. Sex is that thing you only do at night, if you're lucky, or on the sly, or in-between. Confusion abounds.

Why reserve the sense of the erotic for lovers only—for genital sex? What if we came to see our sexuality as the fuel of a healthy life force? What if we understood that the body does more than just egg us on to have sex? Is it conceivable that the sensate messages from the body might be trusty guides? Is it possible that we actually need them for honest communication and connected action? Might the whole of life become more of an erotic experience if we honored the natural and mysterious realm of the sensuous?

An Erotic Relationship with the World

Many years ago, a teacher of mine changed my life when she suggested that just about all human experience, by its very nature, has sexual import; that sexuality, in its broadest sense, means to have a sensual and erotic relationship with the world.

Think about it. We are either initially attracted to or repulsed by people, places, and things. We eventually want to move either toward whatever makes us feel curious and safe, or away from what threatens us. This inborn impulse protects and nurtures us. But when we are forced to compartmentalize sexuality, to separate it from sensuality and touch, we learn to betray who we are. We learn to stop trusting our body selves. We are forced into the habit of living solely from the thinking, visual mind. It's like never allowing your dog off the leash. A dog who never gets to run free in nature, who never gets to smell the smells, bound over fallen trees, and play in the streams, hardly gets to be a real dog. Seeing is not enough. Living life with senses wide open is the key. We need our senses to honor our instincts. They are one of the great miracles of the human design.

When we pay attention to the information we receive through all of our senses, we respond more instinctively and therefore more honestly. When we are living naturally in our bodies, our aesthetic nature is free to enjoy life. Every experience has *physicality*. Space and texture, smell and sound, light and shadow become treasured companions. These qualities evoke powerful feelings like sadness and joy, wonder and comfort. Life has new meaning because it is imbued with feeling and sensation. This makes our "humanness" flourish and evolve. It's like making love to your life.

Try This Now:

Think of yourself as a musical instrument. In order to play well you must be in tune with yourself and with the rest of the orchestra. When you are at the mercy of your neurotic self, you are sharp or flat. Once you know this, you have the choice to get out the tuning fork and bring your tone back to center. When your perfect pitch isn't working, it makes sense to use a tuning fork.

This exercise will help you get in tune physically, emotionally, and mentally—first with yourself, and then with whatever it is that is in front of you. Read the instructions before you do the following exercise. Better yet, ask a friend to read them to you. You may choose to do this exercise with another person, or with any object that attracts you and that you can sense with your entire body—a tree, for example.

> **Stand up and close your eyes.**
>
> **Feel the weight of gravity coming down through your body.**
>
> **Feel your feet on the ground.**
>
> **Relax your jaw, your neck, your buttocks muscles.**
>
> **Take a deep breath in through your nose.**
>
> **Exhale out your mouth with a big sigh.**
>
> **Open your eyes just enough to let in light and shadow, and begin to walk around the room consciously evoking The Posture of Natural Design from Chapter Three.**

Allow yourself to see, hear and sense without naming.

After a few minutes of walking, stop and face your partner, front to front, close but not touching.

Can you face this other and stay present in your body?

Can you feel the entire front of your body as you make contact?

Your face, throat, chest, and belly—your genitals, thighs, knees, lower legs, ankles and feet—without judgment, without thinking in words?

Can you feel the entire front of your body as you make contact?

Do you want to move closer or farther away?

Do you feel safe, curious, awake?

Please don't be polite.

It is far more important to know what your body is really telling you.

Now break your contact.

Walk away and feel the leaving.

What else do you notice?

Walk a few minutes and then find each other again.

This time stand back to back, close but not touching.

Can you feel the entire back of your body as you make contact?

You really do have eyes in the back of your head, in the entire back of your body.

Now break your contact once again.

Walk away and feel the leaving.

Can you feel the sensate print of the other on your body?

> **Are you still present to your sensate experience of the moment?**
>
> **If you are, you are living in your body.**

The body really is smart, a messenger worth heeding. Remember: You can use your senses like a mouth. You can swallow your experiences down into your insides whenever you choose.

Touch Is the Pattern That Connects

Nature is inherently sexual. Have you looked with senses wide open at an orchid or a rose recently? If you enter into what you see, if you use your senses like a mouth, you can "take into yourself" the beauty of a flower in much the same way that you "take in" your lover's sensitive touch through your skin. The act of taking something into yourself makes you feel connected, bonded, and alive. That's why the seeing, hearing, tasting, and sensing of beauty belongs to the realm of the erotic.

Touch is the pattern that connects. At best, it activates the sensation of pleasure, at worst, pain. From the moment of birth, we require loving physical contact with another, body to body. Babies who are deprived of physical contact "fail to thrive"—that is, they die; and prolonged absence of loving touch later in life can make you feel as if life has little meaning. Loving touch that is a natural part of your life can be transformative throughout your life.

Try the exercise you did earlier in this chapter with a prospective lover before you actually engage in lovemaking. If you are willing to heed the messages that your body gives you, I predict that something surprising will happen. You will activate honest and open communication based on the use of all your modes of perception. The decision to have sex with another person is complex. You both deserve the time and energy it takes to stay present emotionally, mentally, and physically, to get to know each other. Well-tuned people can do this because they have consciously worked to train themselves to recognize the right circumstances to make the sexual experience rich and satisfying for both participants. When you are in tune with yourself, you make much better music.

Try This Now:

Ask your partner (this time you need to work with a human) to lie on the floor, face up and eyes closed. Sit beside him or her. Try to let go of all thought by placing attention on sensation, extending unconditional regard to the best of your ability. As you read the following instructions to your partner in a soft, clear voice, remember to stay present in your own body:

> Let your body be heavy, like a rag doll.
>
> Take in a slow deep breath through your nose and let it all out through your mouth with a big sigh.
>
> Relax your face, your jaw, and all of your muscles and joints.
>
> Let the floor support you as you surrender to gravity.
>
> Keep bringing your attention back to sensation.

Now give your partner a minute or two to rest in the instruction. Then,

> Extend your hand and touch your partner with the tips of your index and middle fingers in a nonthreatening place—the front of the shoulder, the middle of the forehead, the bottom of a foot.
>
> Use medium pressure, feeling all the time that your fingertips are connected all the way inside you: to your arm, your shoulder, your chest, and your heart.
>
> Feel the sensation of your fingers as they touch your friend.
>
> What do you notice in the rest of your body?
>
> Can you stay present?
>
> After three or four seconds, take your finger away.

Wait a few moments and touch another spot with the same intentionality and focus. Do this another five or six times, respectfully and randomly. When you are finished, give your partner a moment, and then ask for a report of his or her experience, while keeping his or her eyes closed. You might ask:

> **What are you most aware of right now?**
>
> **Can you feel the print of my finger touches still lingering?**
>
> **How do you feel?**

Ask your partner to open his or her eyes. Sit facing each other and have a conversation about your relationship, while attempting to stay present in your body. Listen with soft eyes, relaxed muscles and an open mind. You might be surprised by what you say, hear, and sense.

The Art of Touch

Touch is a powerful teacher. As the French poet François Fenelon so elegantly says,

> *When you come to be sensibly touched,*
> *the scales will fall from your eyes;*
> *and by the penetrating eyes of love*
> *you will discern that which your other eyes will never see.*

I can tell you from experience that touch can be tricky to teach. So many of us are "touch-phobic" because we are taught early on to believe that touch means sex; and since we are taught that sex is bad, we believe that touch must be bad too. If you have not been touched in a nurturing way for many years, you may not know how to trust yourself or anyone else, how to touch others from a place of unconditional regard. The fact that we live in our precious bodies for years and learn so little about its workings is a sad testament to how estranged we have become from the instinctive part of ourselves.

Most of us are willing to rub another's shoulders; but when we get to the chest and abdomen, well, that's another story. Both giver and receiver start to shut down. Many of my students have told me they are so afraid of puncturing an organ when they start to touch the abdomen of another person that the intimacy involved in this kind of exchange gets lost. Few have ever even pressed on their own bellies to feel what's going on when they have pain or discomfort. Most don't even know where their organs are! This tells me that learning to touch someone must include the study of human anatomy and physiology. It helps to know how the body works and behaves. That way we can concentrate appropriately on the anatomy of intimacy, on the elements of sensation, and put our fearful thinking aside.

As my students experience directly how comforting it is to be deeply touched, even in the more delicate places such as the abdomen and chest, their relationship to just about everything changes. For that reason alone, the study of the art of educated touch is essential. I have seen many hundreds of ordinary folks transform when given the opportunity to experience the giving and receiving of the educated touch of trained human hands. Their relationship to themselves changes because pleasure induction is the true antidote to stress.

John's Story

John's story is a great example of how learning the art of educated touch can change your life for the better. A reserved, well-educated, attractive man in his late thirties, John reported some interesting observations he had made about himself during an ongoing class in educated touch.

Reticently, John confessed that before he enrolled in the program, he related to his body as the "bad" part of himself. He blamed his body for making him think about sex all the time. John hated the fact that every time he saw an attractive woman he would obsessively wonder, "Does she want to have sex with me? Do I want to have sex with her?" If he ever managed to get up the nerve to ask a woman out and eventually have sex with her, he inevitably felt trapped and unfulfilled—afraid of her expectations. Always the "good" boy, he worried that he now owed her his life as proof that he respected her. He walked away from the few relationships he had managed to have hating himself even more.

Through the process of writing his autobiography from the voice of his body, John realized that the adversarial relationship he was having with his instinctive life was due in part to his strict upbringing. He had been marinated in all the fear and loathing of the body that Catholicism often teaches. As a boy he learned to see girls as dangerous because they led a man into sin and temptation. He struggled with whether or not to become a priest. He wanted to be a "good" boy. If that meant willingly relinquishing his sexual life, he would try his best. He wanted to chose the best route to salvation.

Even though this childhood fantasy had long ago been replaced by dreams of family and success—he was now a wealthy executive —John's torturous concerns about what it meant to be a sexual being didn't go away. Consequently, he spent a lot of time alone. He had become a classic workaholic with no wife or family on the horizon. Reality was falling far short of his expectations.

Breathing a sigh of relief, he went on to tell the class that the study of somatics and bodywork had completely changed his worldview. To his amazement he had discovered that he loved the experience of touching others—men or women—from this place the Buddhists call unconditional acceptance. When he removed the possibility of having sex from the situation—not because it was bad or evil, but because it was at cross-purposes from the task at hand—he discovered a well of sensibility and goodwill within himself. He was delightfully freed to engage with his own sensate feedback system. John had finally discovered the elusive key he had been searching for: natural embodiment.

To his great amazement and relief, John found that he no longer wanted to have sex in the same driven way or for the same neurotic reasons. For the first time, that desperate hunting for a sexual partner gave way to a new kind of presence. At long last, he had found the way to real intimacy. He understood that this same awareness could also enhance his sexual experience. He realized what a shame it was to associate the desire to touch and be touched with genital sex alone.

"Touch is really so very much more," he said. "It permeates just about every aspect of our lives. It engenders our sense of warmth and safety. It seems to me that loving touch is essential to our sustained well-being."

The Power of Honest Connection

John was speaking the truth. When we are centered, we have the power to connect honestly, and for the right reasons. The process of touching another while staying connected to our own sensations has the power to unite us. When feelings of control and possession are replaced by a healthy combination of empathy and detachment, we are freed to move toward each other with more openness and interest.

When we close our eyes, center ourselves, and touch another person's body, we can experience what some describe as a "fluid merging." The tissues of the body we are touching gradually become like moist clay on a potter's wheel, or like a swirling energy field alive with spirals and waves. As our attention deepens, we notice changes in our own perception. We can actually feel muscle opening and changing beneath our hands. Our hands become like eyes leading from heart to heart. Our preoccupation with the visual is replaced by the pure, honest joy of sensual pleasure. When we touch or are touched in this way, everyone looks more beautiful. After a good session, both giver and receiver look out of clear eyes that live in a body that is alive in every sense.

My Heart Is in My Hands

Did you know that the hand, especially the thumb, occupies the largest part of the tactile function of motor cortex of the brain? In order to make contact through touch, our hands must be alive. That may sound obvious, but many of us walk around with our brilliant arms and hands swinging lifelessly from our stress-filled shoulders. We hesitate to touch our loved ones because our hands have gone numb.

Try This Now:

> Get up and walk around the room.
>
> Notice how you carry your arms and hands.
>
> Notice that your hands are connected to your wrists,
>   your wrists are connected to your lower arms,

elbows, upper arms—to your shoulders, to the back and front of your chest, to the place where your heart beats and your lungs expand and contract.

Now, imagine that each of your hands is holding a four-inch jar by its top.

Keeping your arms at your sides, with elbows and wrists straight but not locked, quickly rotate your hands in and out, your fingers holding onto the imaginary jar, for about thirty seconds.

This movement will energize your hands, arms and shoulders.

Walk around again feeling how much more alive your hands feel.

Next, bring your hands together in front of you, palm to palm, about four inches apart.

Close your eyes.

Keep your hands there for a while attending to sensation.

Can you feel some heat building?

Move your hands around slowly, keeping them always a small distance away from each other, like they were having a conversation.

Keep bringing your attention back to sensation.

Can you feel more heat and energy growing between your hands?

Play around with this for five minutes or so.

Your hands will feel like they have a mind of their own.

They are like little X-ray machines that can see past skin and reach into the places where tension lives.

They have the power to touch and release this built-up tension.

Your hands are wonderful tools. Don't just let them hang there unnoticed and unused! Live in them, and they will show you how to play a most beautiful instrument: the human body. Now reach out and touch someone else.

Continue this exercise with a partner:

Do the above exercise with a partner.

After you feel the heat building between your own hands, and your partner has too, face each other and put your hands together, palm to palm, keeping them about two inches apart.

Don't talk with words.

Let your eyes be soft and open.

Move together slowly in an under-the-water sort of way, without touching.

Keep the rest of your body alert but relaxed.

Let the rest of your body move if that feels right.

The main thing is to keep your attention focused on sensation.

Feel the heat building in the space between your hands and the hands of your partner.

Let yourself speak the language of the body.

When you're connected, there is no need for a leader or a follower.

Sensation becomes your brightest lantern.

Continue as long as you feel comfortable.

Let the sensations that your body is sending move you.

And Then, Try This:

> Stretch out your arms, palms up, as if you are beckoning a child or a loved one to come to you.
>
> Imagine that your arms are like a garden hose filled with the water of sensation.
>
> This is the universal gesture of connection.
>
> When your arms feel like this, they have what the martial artists call extension.

In order for us to feel connected, to be "well and properly touched" by others and by all of life, all of our perceptions need to be working in concert. When this happens, we feel alive all of the time. We can trust ourselves more because we know in our bodies when to run and when to fight, when to stay and talk, when to stay and make love. The mind can be slippery, but the body seldom lies!

When you are done, take some time to have a verbal conversation about how you each feel—about what you each noticed—about how you are doing. Isn't it a refreshing pleasure to have an embodied conversation?

CHAPTER 6

Be As You Really Are

I laugh when I hear that the fish in the water is thirsty.
You don't grasp the fact that what is most alive of all
is inside your own house.

—KABIR

Before we end Part One and go more deeply into balancing body, mind, and heart in Part Two, we need to do one more step of preparation: We need to awaken what I call the *fair witness,* that intelligence that lives within each of us and observes life and ourselves dispassionately, objectively, and with true-seeing eyes.

Seeing ourselves as we really are is one of the most difficult things we are called to do. That's why, in Chapter Four, I recommend working with a trained somatic educator. In the beginning of our journey, we need a trusty guide to help us hone the skills of honest self-observation. With practice we will eventually be able to guide ourselves.

Years ago, when I first began teaching creative movement classes to three year olds, I would call them into a circle at the end of class and we would sing "Ring Around the Rosy" and all fall down. First, however, I would usually say something like, "Take a moment and look at all the faces in this circle, look at how different we all are, isn't it wonderful?" We would all look around and marvel. And then one day one of the children stopped me in my tracks when he said, "But Johanna, I can't see my own face!"

I didn't know what to say. As I remember, I laughed, and we all fell down. Later I thought to myself, "Get used to it kid. You'll never get to see your own face, and it will make you crazy for the rest of your life."

The cruelest cosmic joke of all is that you get to see me and I don't. That goes for you too, you know! I see me reflected in your face. You see you reflected in mine. When we like the reflection we see, we feel good. When we don't, we go searching for a better friend. We place our worth, along with our attention, on our own biased interpretation of a mere reflection.

The Face in the Mirror

It all goes back to Narcissus, the strikingly handsome young man of Greek mythology who saw his own reflection in a deep clear pool and fell hopelessly in love—with himself. He is the classic archetype depicting self-fascination and self-absorption: the icon of our age.

Narcissus, the son of the river god Cephissus, was so extraordinarily beautiful that every nymph who saw him fell in love with him on sight. But he was so vain that he regularly spurned their advances. Then Echo, the fairest of the nymphs, fell in love with Narcissus. Unfortunately, because of a curse placed on her by the powerful goddess Hera for talking too much, she was doomed to be able to repeat only what was spoken to her. She followed Narcissus everywhere, hiding behind trees and bushes waiting for the right time to be seen by him.

One day, when he was separated from a group of his friends while playing in the woods, she had her chance. Narcissus heard the rustle of some bushes nearby and called out, "Who's here?"

"Here," Echo called.

"Then come" said Narcissus.

"Come." she cried.

"Leave your hiding place," said Narcissus, "and we'll play."

"We'll play," she called, as she happily ran to embrace him.

Narcissus backed away in horror, saying, "I'd rather die than let you touch me."

Echo was so humiliated by the cruel refusal of her love that she hid in a cave and wasted away until nothing was left of her but her voice.

To punish Narcissus, the avenging goddess Nemesis set a trap. One day, while hunting in the mountains, Narcissus came across a pool of clear water. Leaning over to drink from it, he saw his own beautiful reflection. Instantly entranced, he believed he was seeing the spirit who lived in the pool. As he admired the beauty of the face reflected back at him, Narcissus fell hopelessly in love. He bent to kiss the image. He reached to embrace it. But whenever he touched the water, the image would disappear. Heartbroken, Narcissus stayed by the pool weeping, until his beauty faded and he died.

The body of Narcissus was never found. All that remained was a flower, purple within and surrounded by white petals, drooping over its own reflection in the pool.

Poor Narcissus! He fell in love with a two-dimensional—that is, unembodied—image. He got locked in the visual mode, attaching his projected dreams and desires to his own image. No one had warned him that seeing with the eyes alone is not enough. No one had touched him in the way that awakens pleasure and empathy. As the inspired Sufi poet Kabir profoundly says in the verse that begins this chapter, "What is most alive of all is *inside* your own house."

Narcissism is what happens when we shut down our senses, our ability to reach outside of ourselves and sense what it is like to walk in someone else's shoes. When we believe that our view of the world is the absolute truth, when we insist on seeing others as two-dimensional reflected images, as part of our mirror, we suffer like Narcissus. We suffer because we project onto the others in our lives our hopes, our dreams, and our fears, unconsciously making them mere actors in our little drama. The cruel joke is that neither of us knows it! The following true story is an endearing illustration of how we "make each other up," and how little our story has to do with the truth.

Jason's Story

When he was in his late twenties, my good friend Jason signed up for a ten-day meditation retreat. Tall, dark, and handsome, rich and well-educated, he was smitten with spirituality and imagined himself to be ripe for enlightenment. He figured that surely within ten days he could learn to erase all of his ego hang-ups by practicing detached acceptance of all suffering. He would then go on to achieve a state of divine grace.

The meditation retreat was conducted in silence. There would be no socializing, no TV, radio, reading, or phone calls. Each person was asked instead to use every aspect of their time to pay fair witness attention to their own process.

More than 100 people participated in the retreat. All willingly sat cross-legged and straight-backed on pillows for forty-five minutes at a time. Then they walked consciously for twenty minutes, attending to the sensation of every aspect of the walking process. Then they sat again. The instructions were to simply place attention on the sensation of breath inhaled thorough the nose. When the mind started thinking about something, or the body hurt or itched, or when there was some distracting noise in the room, you were to kindly call your attention back to the sensation of breath, period. No melodrama, no judgment, no excuses.

On the first day, Jason was ecstatic. He gave himself an "A" in meditation. Enlightenment was close at hand! Meditation was a piece of cake. Maybe his karma was to become a holy monk on the path. The first few hours of the next day passed quickly. Then he noticed the woman sitting just four people down and to the right.

She was elegant, beautiful. The afternoon light illuminated her face and hands in an enchanting way. It was love at first sight. Jason had finally seen the woman of his dreams, and all he could think about was how he would make love to her, how he would care for her, how he would propose to her. When the voice of his fair witness suggested gently that he bring his attention back to the sensation of breath, his ego was quick to say explicitly, "You don't understand. I have just met 'the one.' There is nothing more important than that. I must get to know her. I will!"

And so he did—in his mind. His newly met fair witness disappeared as he completely gave way to his ego-driven imagination. He saw the house she grew up in, met her parents, introduced her to his, and gallantly spirited her away to the most idyllic place, where they made mad, passionate love and he told her his deepest secrets. She understood him perfectly. She was his muse, his angel, his soulmate.

On the fourth day of the retreat, however, she began to bore him. Her hair wasn't quite right, she seemed a bit depressed, unassertive, even ordinary. He ended the relationship and chastised himself for getting diverted. He willed himself to bring his attention back to more important things, like the sensation of breath and his own enlightenment. Thank God he could now enjoy a few blissful moments and get back on the path.

That evening, during the last hour of meditation, Jason noticed yet another beautiful woman. He dreamed about her in the night, and the next day was convinced that yes, this was really the elusive "one." Once again, he could not pull his mind away from her. He fell in love, got disappointed and bored, ended the relationship, and with great indignation, returned to seeking nirvana—all during the meditation session. Much to his dismay (and his credit), he realized that his neurotic mind was just about completely out of control.

At the end of the retreat, even Jason could see that he was far away from enlightenment. Much to his embarrassed amazement, he realized that his imaginary experiences at the retreat reflected the story of all his actual relationships with women. It was as though they were never really there. All had been eclipsed by the expectations of his own imagination. Once a woman spoke outside the script he had unconsciously given her, he ended the relationship dispassionately, saying mean things like, "I'm sorry, you're just not 'the one.' I just can't commit to someone like you."

This realization shocked Jason into reality. He was now willing to explore the trap of his own narcissistic demands. As the Sufis say, "Once the magician shows you the trick, it isn't magic anymore." Jason got himself into therapy soon after that. He began to examine his life's assumptions and face the truth about himself.

Take Away the Mirror

It is time for all of us who are mesmerized by our own two-dimensional reflection in the mirror to wake up, break the trance of our narcissism, and return to a more sensate relationship with the world around us. It is time to feel our connection to all things. It is time for us to open our senses. In order to do this, we must awaken our fair witness, building an alliance between what the ego-driven mind imagines and what actually *is*—between our ego's desires and the needs of the whole ecosystem, from which we are inseparable.

"Mirror, Mirror On the Wall . . . ?"

We get little encouragement from society at large to break the mirror. In fact, we get asked all the time to buy *more* mirrors. Our cultural narcissism is so powerful that we have created a billion-dollar fitness industry and a multibillion-dollar movie and fashion industry to keep it in place. We regularly worship at the feet of the great mythic, mind-perfected appearance body. We insist on modeling ourselves on airbrushed photographs of people who pretend to be just like us, on people who have spent thousands surgically acquiring perfect teeth and noses and breasts.

The "ordinary" people (that is, most of us) feel profoundly isolated in our imagined "defectiveness." We worry that if we gain five pounds, or get wrinkles, or smell bad, our perfect beloved will leave us for another. Sometimes this really happens because people believe their partner's appearance will reflect back on them. Many abandon their so-called significant others because they have nothing to exchange but their "appearance selves" and their inflated dreams of the perfect relationship.

More and more, people outside the entertainment industry are investing in their appearance: plastic surgery, hair implants, home gym equipment, diet bars, personal trainers. Young women are getting breast implants as high school graduation gifts, middle-aged executives are getting facelifts to keep up with their younger competition. Yet, despite all this concern with how we appear to others, we are strangely out of touch with our bodies and our senses. On top of that we are a culture of people who are actually fearful about touching each other, body to body. We'd rather have phone-sex or cyber-sex.

We are quickly forgetting how to separate the dream from reality. In fact we seem to value our dreams more. After all, one must be much more careful about what happens body to body—about what you learn through direct experience. We are warned that too much interest in the experience of the senses leads to hedonism, to danger, to disease, to death.

So, rather cruelly, our society enforces both our fascination with the body and our alienation from it. Hard to imagine that awareness and discipline are required to really participate in the realm of the senses. And so we worship physical fitness and perfection instead.

When We See Life in Our Own Image

When image means more to us than who we actually are—than the process of becoming human—we are in deep trouble. That, combined with our need to be the best through doing the most, has left many feeling empty, afraid of the silence of being. We compensate for this repression of instinct by blatantly refusing to explore the possibility that our precious thinking might be skewed—that miscommunication stems partly from our tendency to "make each other up," as Jason did, to suit our needs and prove our theories.

We seem to have convinced ourselves that speaking mind to mind is communication enough, that Webster's definitions give the real meaning, that body language needs no dictionary. But take a moment to think about it this way: We learn to speak the language of our family of origin first, the language of our motherland second, and the language of our friends and lovers when we are lucky. The fact that we speak English (or whatever language you were born speaking) to each other in every case confuses us deeply. The variations on meaning boggle mind and heart and body.

For example, in my family anger was taboo. We had to go to our room until we could speak rationally and politely. When one of my best friends yelled at me for what she experienced as withholding love, I thought I'd die. In my family she would have been excommunicated for such behavior. The only way I knew to react was to go to my room and never speak to her again. She, on the other hand, was raised in a family where the expression of anger was the norm. Everyone yelled at each other when they were angry and frustrated. It was the only way to survive.

Even though this incident happened long after I had left home and was living on my own, I automatically turned on my heel and walked away. I was thinking, "That's it. You're history. Our friendship is over." This was not acceptable behavior in my world. If only she could say the same words without yelling. If only she would control herself and speak the language of my family. Then I could continue to be her friend.

At the time I didn't know that I had such a strict set of rules and expectations. I didn't even know (and would have adamantly denied) that I was angry back. So it made sense that I couldn't understand why some of my friends accused me of being conditional and intimidating. I didn't know how frightened I was of becoming anything other than what my family had programmed me to be. I didn't know that other software was available for my hard drive to read.

Luckily for me, I listened when my friend followed me to my room saying, "You can leave if you want, but you can also stay. Can't you see that I'm angry at you because I care? I don't want you to go. I want you to give me more of yourself. I want to feel your passion. Don't make me the bad guy. We can work this out." I was deeply touched. For the first time I got to see and feel that there was another way of communicating. My family's way was not the only way. I realized that I had a lot to learn—that there was more to heartfelt communication than I had ever imagined.

The fact that we tend to view ourselves and our friends through "family of origin" blinders goes a long way toward explaining why we keep being "surprised" by life over and over again. We can't understand why that perfect lover who said all the right things turned out to be "such a heart breaker," why that perfect couple down the street suddenly got an acrimonious divorce, why that boss who seemed so willing to embrace me in the corporate family turned out to be "such a dictator."

Why do we keep making the same mistakes about people over and over? Why do we behave the way we do? One theory holds that personality is a defense (mental, emotional, and physical) against childhood wounding and therefore not the true self. Unless we are shown otherwise, personality only knows how to communicate in family of origin dialect or in reaction to family of origin dialect. One might think of personality as protective suiting—like the bumper of a car, designed to take the blows while protecting the essential structure of the psyche. We all know that it's essential to wear a padded uniform while playing football. However, no one warns us that when you come home at the end of a hard day and get in bed with your lover, you should be able to take your protective uniform off.

Unfortunately, many of us can't. Our personality has become our uniform, and we've forgotten that we weren't born wearing it. The consequences are devastating. Our capacity for intimacy is hampered when we can't ever reveal our nakedness—when we can't honor our senses, when we can't feel, body to body, that we are all connected.

More than we are willing to admit, we are the product of our own biased programming. I expect you to understand me. I move toward you if I imagine you do understand me, away from you if I imagine you don't. The problem is, I don't think I'm imagining. I am a shrewd lawyer for my own concerns. I can interpret the law to suit my own needs and not even realize it.

We are caught between outdated yet powerful cultural rules, our repressed natural instincts, the language of our family of origin, and our sincere desire to become conscious. Just as the beautiful Narcissus of Greek mythology was trapped by his enchantment with his own reflection in the lake, we are caught in the trap of our own self-serving worldview, which urges us to stare only at our reflected image while failing to develop an inner life.

What does it take to see that our perception of reality is biased, that we are not allowing our bodies, hearts, and minds to report accurately? Are we doomed to be in constant reaction to our own projections and not even know it? How can we begin the work of examining what is really inside so we can truly see what is outside?

Breaking the Trance of Narcissus: Developing Your Fair Witness

"And if I die before I wake . . ." We're all familiar with that time-worn traditional bedtime prayer. An old Sufi saying adds a startling dimension: "*Must* I die before I wake?" Fortunately, no.

We develop an inner life by learning how to disengage willingly from our habits of body, heart, and mind—by practicing a more unbiased way of perceiving. This process teaches us how we can explore empathy, first for ourselves, and then rippling outward to include others.

Many spiritual traditions recommend cultivating an internalized "fair witness" as a way to find peace. That means being willing to find the impartial voice inside yourself and place it in between your most nagging critical voice and your most inflated grandiose voice.

The fair witness voice is willing to relinquish control and allow outcome. It interrupts the ongoing war between our various selves, the war that deadens the body and confuses the mind. It is way better than drugs and alcohol!

The fair witness helps evoke the sense of center by maintaining an open attention that chooses acceptance over resignation, sensation over flawed thinking and feeling. It watches over our ego's contradictions and helps us not take ourselves quite so seriously. Fair witness attention cultivates and enhances the state of relaxed wakefulness. This simple meditation is the best way I've found in day-to-day life of developing a knowing that is not so controlled by ego-centered concerns—by a personal bias based on ignorance, fear, confusion, and the need to always be "right."

Dan Rather Meets My Fair Witness

For reasons I've never been able to figure out, I call the voice of my narcissistic or not-so-fair witness "Dan Rather." He is always reporting on my behavior and the behavior of those around me, whether I ask him to or not. He relentlessly reports on how I'm faring. He tells me who is better than I am, how I am losing, how I am stupid, superior, or overlooked. He is a busy-body, a hateful gossip who keeps me agonizingly self-conscious, self-serving, and self-righteous —not to mention anxious, shy, and distrustful. He rudely breaks in on what peace of mind I do manage to have, reminding me of what is missing, how lazy I am, and what I have to do next. Embarrassingly, I am compelled to tune into his show every day, come rain or shine.

For years I bought into his trenchant opinions hook, line, and sinker. His relentless criticism wreaked havoc on my self-esteem and drained my emotional bank account. Then, with the help of my teachers, I discovered the voice of my fair witness. As I learned how to tune into that voice, which, it turns out, was inside me all along, I willingly gave her the power to interrupt Dan. To my delight, my internal life got a beautiful makeover. Now when Dan starts haranguing, she calmly tells him to be quiet.

Then she reminds me to breathe deeply as I shift my attention to sensation. She encourages me to extend unconditional regard to all beings, to stay my course. When I am willing to listen, I trust myself more. I feel calmer and more connected to what is actually happening.

My fair witness also tells me when I am inappropriately living in the past, or living it out over and over again. She knows that over-reactive thinking and feeling on my part usually means I am once again at the mercy of the unresolved disappointments from my past. When I can make room to listen during those times of crisis, my fair witness diplomatically reminds me that my resentment only poisons me—that I can choose to stop the chatter of my old melodrama tape and center myself in my body by seeing, hearing, and sensing what is true in my world *right now*.

My fair witness knows when I am thinking emotionally rather than clearly. She knows that distorted emotionality only gives me more reasons not to move forward, toward what I really want. She is hip to Dan's sneaky ways, his technique of drawing my attention to what is missing, to how unfair life can be, to plain old obsessive worry and conjecture. When Dan is in control, I am predictably off course.

Tuning In to Your Fair Witness

In some ways, your mind is like a radio. You can press the button to change the channel. Your attention is what gives you the ability to see the button—to reach out with mindfulness and change the channel accordingly. One of life's dirty tricks is that all the channels play simultaneously (even though we hear only one at a time): the news channel keeps you informed, the classical music channel makes you feel relaxed, the rock channel energized, the talk channel a part of the human condition. Reality changes when you change the channel.

The "neurotic mind" is like the talk show channel, full of judgments and melodrama. The fair witness channel is the one that plays peaceful sounds twenty-four hours a day—waves gently lapping on the shore, the wind blowing over the ridgeline, the brook bubbling over smooth stones. It calms you down so you can see and feel and be more honest. To feel centered, all you have to do is learn how to change channels. It's really pretty simple once you get the hang of it. Unfortunately, simple doesn't necessarily mean easy. It takes practice to stay centered, especially when the winds of crisis knock us around.

The next time you're caught in emotional and mental gridlock, try changing the channel. Listen to the waves breaking on the beach for a while and then come back to your dilemma. This simple practice can help you to let go of the ego's negative, obsessive, useless, and inaccurate imagining and get back to a less attached position. This allows body, heart, and mind to get in tune with each other. When that happens, life is much easier to navigate.

The first step is to admit to the limitations of your own narcissism. Once you see that your real self has been in a war waged between the contradictory messages that come from egoistic thoughts, sensations, and feelings—between the past and the present—you can relax, sit back in your own skin and bones, and respond to life with more ease, freedom, and appropriateness. You can stop your constant, defensive reactivity and finally see what *is*. This is an integral step to paving the way for more honest and fulfilling relationships.

When Jason realized the power of his narcissistic imagination, he was appalled. When he called and asked for some advice, I told him about the following exercise, which I call "I See, I Feel, I Imagine." The goal is learning to tell the difference between seeing, feeling, and imagining.

Try This Now:

> Pick out a person, place, or thing and simply see it.
>
> Report exactly what you see.
>
> Eliminate all judgments and interpretations, likes or dislikes.
>
> Just stick to the facts, ma'am.
>
> Now, look again.
>
> Notice how seeing triggers feelings.
>
> Next, look again.
>
> Notice how seeing triggers imagination.

Does that seem too easy? Here's an example of what may be going on in your mind:

"As I look at my friend, I see that his hair and eyes are brown. I see that he is wearing a red T-shirt. I see that the wall behind him is painted blue. Period. I am reporting exactly what I see. I choose to eliminate all judgments and interpretations, likes or dislikes. Just stick to the facts, ma'am.

"When I look again, paying attention to my feelings, it goes like this: I see your brown eyes and hair, and I feel envious. Your red shirt makes me feel pleased. It is the perfect shade of red. The blue wall behind you wrecks everything. It reminds me of my mother's house and I feel alienated.

"When I look with my imagination, it goes like this: I see your brown hair and eyes and I imagine that you admire yourself regularly. I assume that your mother really loved and supported you, that, unlike me, you had a wonderful childhood. I imagine that your ex-girl friend gave you that shirt for your birthday. The fact that you still wear it means that you have not let go of that relationship. You are not really available. You've been leading me on. I shut down and pull away."

And so it goes. More than we like to admit, I believe my own imaginings without checking them out with you. Even more embarrassing is that I might believe my imagination *even when you tell me a different story.*

The real goal is to learn how to tell the difference between our natural intuition or gut sense and our own biased projections. That is the goal of this exercise. Seeing what actually is cleans the palate. It is a relief simply to see. To be present. To take responsibility for your own assumptions. Your friends will feel the difference in how you relate to them. All of us want to be accepted for who we are. All of us want to be given the chance and the choice to change—to actively heal our personalities.

PART TWO

The Art and
Practice
of Living
in Your Body

CHAPTER 7

Creating the Body–Heart–Mind Connection

> Am I willing to give up what I have in order to be
> what I am not yet?
> Am I willing to let my ideas of myself, of humanity
> be changed?
>
> —M. C. RICHARDS

As you saw in Part One, our bodies are continually sending us fundamental information about our environment and our well-being that our neurotic minds unconsciously choose to ignore, embellish, control, or misinterpret:

> You shake hands with a stranger, warmth and kinship seem to flow into you. Your heart and body say, *Pursue this relationship.* Your suspicious mind tells you, *I must be imagining things,* and makes your body turn away.

> You walk home at night, and you get a feeling in your belly that says, *Run!* Your controlling mind says, *You wimp, get it together. Everything is fine.* One block later you are robbed. Your mind wonders, *How did my body know I was in danger?*

You go on a long walk and return home feeling fit and refreshed. Your body says, *That feels great.* But when you look in the mirror through the filter created by an envious heart, your judgmental mind says, *You'll never look the way you should.* The result: You continue to *feel* inadequate, resentful, and depressed.

You pass a bakery and the smell of chocolate calls to every cell of your body. Your body says, *Just a little chocolate would make me feel great right now.* Your self-righteous mind tells your "greedy" body, *You have absolutely no self-control.* At home, you make yourself eat a carrot. Your mind feels victorious but that doesn't keep the rest of you from feeling miserable.

Your lover's touch feels rough and insensitive. Your muscles tense up and you can't seem to get in a romantic mood. Your body and heart say, *We really don't like the way this feels.* Your mind says, *There must be something wrong with me.* Guilty thinking convinces you to have sex anyway. You numb your discomfort by visualizing someone else. The next day your mind can hardly remember whether you had sex or not. You can't understand why you feel so out of sorts.

Why Don't We Listen?

Every child is taught (even though the body is programmed to figure it out anyway) to heed the messages the tangible environment sends the body: The stove is hot—don't touch. It's snowing out—wear a jacket. This food tastes good—eat it. Learning to listen to these messages and interpret them correctly ensures our survival.

At the same time the body is also sending messages about its feelings and perceptions of the less tangible world. Unfortunately, these are the messages we are taught to discount early on. Deep down, we feel we should pay attention to these signals, but we think we must reject them as dangerous and untrustworthy. So instead of including the wisdom of our natural biology as part of life's equation, we choose to listen almost exclusively to the voice of our ego-driven culturally civilized rational mind, or our ego-driven culturally overreactive irrational emotions, or our out-of-balance overstressed sensory input—and then wonder why we don't feel more at home in the world.

One fact we are seldom taught at school (or even in our family of origin) is that from birth we have three primary ways of perceiving and interpreting the messages that come to us: with the *belly* center, the home of sensation; with the *heart* center, the home of emotions; and with the *head* center, the home of thought. Each center has its own intelligence, language, type of intuition, and terrain; each center is influenced by the others; each center can lead or follow; and each center can be forced out of balance by life's bumps and turns. Our interaction with both the internal and external worlds around us is driven by the interplay between these three centers of perception. The problem is that the centers frequently contradict each other —your body says "Leave this relationship, it makes me tense"; your heart says "I'm in love, I can't help it"; your head says "Stay, you've got financial security. Where are you going to go?" The result is that we feel frustrated and perplexed. To get relief from our confusion, we often decide to heed the input from primarily one center. We may feel better in the moment, but we are bound to feel more confusion later on.

Most of us end up trapped in one perceptual center, thinking we are perceiving what really happened. We listen to our belly, our heart, or our head, depending on which center we've given our lives to. This is the human situation depicted so profoundly in Akira Kurosawa's classic film *Rashomon*. In this film, each witness to an event is asked to relate his or her story of what happened. The stories roll out, each person's perception radically different from the others. Which is the most true? Like the characters in *Rashomon,* your centers are all together when they perceive an event. But when asked to report what happened, they each can tell a startlingly different story.

The famous east Indian legend of the six blind men and the elephant is another example. Six blind men are asked to inspect an elephant and then describe the creature. The first happens to fall against the elephant's side and imagines him to be like a wall. The second, feeling only the tusk, fancies this very same animal to be just like a spear. The third, taking hold of the trunk, thinks the elephant to be like a snake. The fourth, touching the knee, imagines a tree. The fifth, stroking an ear, feels a fan. The sixth, taking hold of the tail, imagines the elephant to be like a rope. Each was partly right, and all were wrong. Sensation alone is not enough to provide a complete picture.

Most people smile and nod their heads in recognition when they hear this paradoxical teaching parable. More often than not, reality seems to be in the eye of the beholder and that fact has caused us all a lot of distress. It's easy enough to find examples outside the realm of film and parable. Just ask any divorced couple what (or who) caused their marriage to disintegrate. I guarantee you'll get two different stories.

So, before we go any further, let's take a look at the nature of the three centers of perception. Each description is loosely drawn, thought provoking, and certainly not meant to be set in stone. The trouble with categorizing behavior is that there are always exceptions. Please don't take this too literally. You might try listening with each of your centers of perception wide open before you decide the truth of the matter. Use these descriptions as a creative tool to strengthen your "fair witness," as a way to have more of yourself to live your life with. What's drawn here is simply an attempt to illustrate and honor the mysterious complexity of the anatomy of perception—how and why we suffer from being only partly right—and to provide a useful map to follow on the road to becoming a decent human being.

For real-life unadulterated examples of how the centers work in tandem, go to a playground and watch children under the age of three freely displaying the power of these natural resources. When children fall down they usually get right back up and try again. When they are having a good time their voices sing out with pleasure. When they hurt their voices alert us to their pain. They primarily let their bodies lead the way into each experience. Their natural sense of balance is a wonder to behold.

The challenge, of course, is to integrate all the contradictions into a unified whole, where the right side knows what the left is doing and vice versa, where conscious awareness and natural embodiment can walk together hand in hand.

The Belly Center: Our Gut Instinct

The belly center is the home of our gut instinct, the place that speaks the language of sensation. When our belly center is functioning properly, it tells us when we are feeling cold or hot, pain or pleasure, tired or awake, scared or safe, hungry or well-fed, aroused or angry. It is the home of our territorial responsiveness. It governs how we relate to the physical world around us. It automatically tells us when the chairs are comfortable, when the dinner smells good, when the bed sheets need washing, where we want to sit at the restaurant, where we draw the line.

However, in the West, we let the rules of "polite society" shape our movements. Women learn to cross their legs when they sit, even when it becomes uncomfortable to do so. Men learn to move with stiff, "macho" mannerisms of one degree or another. We rarely see natural movement in others, let alone in ourselves.

Every once in a while, we are fortunate to glimpse natural movement captured on film. A comic movie from the early 1980s, *The Gods Must Be Crazy,* featured the San tribe of Africa's Kalahari Desert, a people who lived in harmony with their environment. In the film we are able to see that the bodies of the adults are as supple as their children, their smiles as genuine. They move with untarnished grace and natural intelligence. Clearly, they are in touch with their inborn sense of direction, space, and timing. They are not living an *idea* of what they think their bodies should look like, they *are* their bodies. It is plain to see how these people live in harmony with themselves, with nature, with Earth's body.

The Heart Center:
How We Feel About the World

The heart center is the home of our emotions, the place that speaks the language of feeling, the place that gives meaning to life. If it's functioning properly, emotion tells us when we feel mad, sad, bad, or glad; loved or rejected; attached, blamed, abandoned, or forgiving. It compels us to reach out and make contact with others. It tells us when our lover is aroused, when our children are hurting, when we want to throw our arms around a friend, or when to wail in grief. It is the home of our bonding response. It governs how we feel about the world. It automatically tells us who to love and who to hate, what is beautiful and what is ugly. It is the perception that allows us to be moved to tears. We need emotion to thrive and prosper.

Emotion is what connects us to nature and all living things. Nature and music both have the power to evoke deep feeling. They have the power to tear open the hearts of even the most shut down of people. The sound of violins pulls on our heart strings and helps us release our grief. The glory of a sunrise can raise our spirits up and fill our hearts with joy.

We see the heart center function most naturally in very young children. Expressing their feelings is the most natural thing in the world for them—and we respond. When they cry, we feel compelled to pick them up; when they smile, we smile back without thinking. Children are innocent and unselfconscious; they won't be denied. They are unified with feeling.

That's why many among our adult population have been on a collective search for the elusive (sometimes irritating) "inner" child. They want to be able to authentically express their feelings and still be taken seriously by the others in their lives. They have an over-powering longing to genuinely love and be loved. However, some of us can get lost in the longing to return to the innocence of child-hood and mistakenly celebrate all emotional expression as honest interaction.

There is a world of difference between feeling and hysteria, be-tween feeling deeply and acting out or throwing a tantrum. Emotion is not by nature loud and in your face. When it is grounded and honest, emotion can be subtle and profound or all-consuming. How-ever, when we give up this understanding in favor of "correct," con-trolled behavior, we can get caught in the limitations of adulthood. Our natural feeling of innocence can only survive when an honest, open heart is combined with a balanced body and mind. This wise old Sufi proverb says it best: "The unconflicted state of the baby is not the unconflicted state of the guru."

The Head Center:
How We Think About the World

The head center is the home of our thoughts, rational and otherwise; the place that translates those thoughts into words and visual images. When functioning properly, it governs our curiosity, our desire to understand where we come from, why we're here and what the universe is about in all its awesome glory. The mind is analytic. It wants to know the facts, to analyze the data, to get ahead through thinking. The head center wants to understand the universe, to talk directly with the gods, "to go where no man (or woman) has ever gone before." We call mind *egotistic* when we use it only in our own best interests, when it has the power to block the felt experience of body states such as empathy and compassion. We call it *enlightened* when it works in tandem with healthy instinct and emotion.

The head center controls how we *think* about the world. It plans for the future, remembers the past, invents new products, and discovers the unknown. It figures things out. It is our culture's designated policeman of instinct because it can both create and remember the rules. It has the power to overrule emotions and sensations and is the genius child of Western civilization. It is the jewel in the crown of humankind. Descartes' conclusion that "I think, therefore I am" makes us feel superior to all other animals. Both the positive and negative consequences of this two-dimensional view of the world are plain to see.

Some speculate that the mind is the main source of our fear of living—that the inability to understand the real meaning of life, combined with childhood trauma, scares us out of our bodies into a highly intelligent mind that we hope can figure out why we're here and how to keep us safe. Our knowledge that death and taxes are inevitable puts us into a permanent state of dread, and gives fearful thoughts the power to activate the body's fight/fight instinct.

Once activated in this way, we continue the process because we *think* we have the power to figure out where the next life-threatening

danger is going to come from—that the head center alone can determine how to deal with our concerns about the things that might be-
fall us. And sometimes our defensive thinking saves us. The problem
is that thoughts without sensation are only two-dimensional and, for
that reason, often inaccurate. We can think ourselves into a permanent state of stress when everything around us is actually fine. We
can also think ourselves into a permanent state of optimism when
everything around us is actually falling apart.

Sometimes "using your head" isn't enough. We need to access
feeling and sensation together with thinking in order to perceive life
in three dimensions.

Seeking Balance

Experience won't register on the bones and muscles, let alone
the heart, unless the body is hooked up. In fact, when we lose conscious perception of body input, we are likely to suffer from an am-
nesia of actual experience. When we organize our attention around
ideas that are essentially designed to protect us from danger, or to
generate hope and self-importance, we become hypersensitive, over-
alert, and grandiose. We can even become aversive to touch, to too
much human contact in general. This is because our muscles have
to be on guard and ready to fight or run at all times.

Since fear and pleasure cannot exist simultaneously in a healthy
organism, pleasure that leads to bonding gets sacrificed. Those who
are stuck in thought must re-learn how to turn off the fight/flight reflex. This can only happen when we learn to doubt the fear that originates in the mind and learn to look again, with senses wide open,
trusting instinct as an essential guide.

Instinct combined with clear thinking is what allows us to respond appropriately, without premeditation. When the United States
women's soccer team beat China, every commentator I saw asked
the young woman who kicked the winning goal what she was thinking at that moment. Her reply was immediate: "Absolutely nothing."
She trusted her body and her training to be her guide. The reporters
didn't seem to understand that an over-strategizing stressed-out mind
would have blocked her kick.

The best medicine for curing the situation is the study of awareness. We can learn how to consciously clear our narcissistic habits of body, heart and mind. With interest and training, we can learn to live our lives with clarity, integrity, and compassion.

Learning to use all of our senses means activating our three centers of perception: belly, heart, and mind. Awareness and practice are the two keys that unlock this door.

The fair witness consciousness we explored in Chapter Six is a basic groundwork for a broader perception of reality, but there is more. We must also learn to recognize our conditioned tendency to use one mode of perception in favor of the others. The next three chapters should give you a good idea of where you fall in this spectrum and some steps you can take to get in balance.

As you read, remember: No one is ruled by just one center. We each have our own unique recipes for combining mind, heart, and body. Still, as you read you will recognize the center that prevails right now. That is where you should begin your work.

CHAPTER 8

Opening the Mind

> There exists for all of us, initially, a state of
> precommunication in which our intentions play
> across the body of another, and vice versa.
>
> — MERLEAU-PONTY

Thoughts are powerful.

Have you ever been tormented by the sudden thought that you
were in danger? You felt your heart beating faster, your mouth getting dry, your entire being overcome by the desire to run? Your mind
was sure a robber or a mugger or a mad dog was about to get you—
but nothing happened. No one was there. It was all in your head.
You couldn't sleep for the rest of the night. You were up all night because your mind couldn't turn your body off.

Maybe it happened while you were driving over a bridge. Out of
nowhere, you panicked. Your heart started thumping, your breath was
completely out of control, you broke out in a sweat, you felt like you
would pass out any second. Your mind screamed, "Pull over, you're
having a heart attack, you're going to die!" But you didn't die. You
pulled off the road, somehow got it back together, and realized it was
all in your head.

Have you ever started a relationship and been overtaken by the
thought that it won't work out? Even though you had a great first
date, you're convinced that if you call for another one, you'll be

politely refused. Your stomach is in knots already. Maybe you avoid intimate relationships altogether, feeling much safer having a relationship with the thoughts in your own mind.

Perhaps the major lesson you learned from adolescence was your body wasn't trustworthy, and feelings and sensations were messy and scary and unpredictable. Your mind was a far better place to reside in. There you had almost complete control. No one could get in, and you had a good view of the area. You could fill your mind with all the great ideas of humankind, you could even formulate your own, you could imagine a life far better than the real deal. Having a body and being in physical relationship with others were vastly overrated.

Then one day it dawned on you maybe it was time to have a real relationship. Perhaps you were lonely after all. But no matter how hard you tried, you couldn't quite make contact. Your fear of invasion had blocked your instinctive sense so well you couldn't reach out even when you wanted to. You had no bridge between body, heart, and mind.

If you identify in some way with any of these scenarios, you have put your mind in charge of your body. The reason these are such unsettling experiences is because your body is trying to get your attention!

When the Fight/Flight Response Is Always On

When we are in harm's way—when there's a real threat to our lives—our bodies' fight/flight instinct naturally compels us to fight or flee. Because this response is governed by the sympathetic nervous system, we don't have to think, we don't have to figure anything out, we just respond in the moment to the situation. The brain cries "Danger!"; the adrenal glands pump adrenaline through the bloodstream to give us the speed and strength we need to survive; the heart beats faster to make sure the blood gets where it's most needed; and we breathe faster so we get enough oxygen to keep it all going. What happens? Miracles. We lift the car off the baby, run faster than we ever imagined to escape the forest fire, jump into the lake and swim half a mile to save a drowning child.

Some people, however, have an unconscious habit of substituting fearful, obsessive thinking for the body's natural intelligence. Where instinct once responded appropriately to danger, a fearful mind now is responsible for chronic anxiety in the body. The adrenaline keeps pumping, the heart beats wildly, and we can't seem to get a good breath. It's as if the red alert button gets stuck in the "on" position.

In his book *Why Zebras Don't Get Ulcers: A Guide to Stress, Stress-Related Diseases, and Coping,* Stanford University professor Robert M. Sapolsky presents an intriguing case for the idea that people develop many diseases partly because the body is not designed to endure a lifestyle that causes constant stress—an abusive home life, sitting in daily traffic jams, or working overtime chasing unreasonable deadlines. Rather, like other mammals, humans are built for the kind of short-term stress faced by a zebra—like outrunning a lion. When a zebra narrowly escapes from the jaws of death, he doesn't have to get into psychotherapy in order to get over the trauma. The next day the zebra is back to normal, trusting instinct to tell him when the lion is sleeping and when the lion is on the hunt.

When we live with ongoing, continual stress, especially during the formative years, the body responds as if we were in danger: It produces too much adrenaline. Too much adrenaline causes the mind to think fearfully, fear blocks the pleasure response and puts us in a bind: We can't use pleasure as a way to calm down and assess the situation. This makes it very difficult to manage stress, to know the difference between fantasy and reality, to live comfortably in our bodies. It is mind over matter all the way: "I think, therefore I am."

When the Narcissistic Mind Is in Charge, Fear Rules the Body

If you are mind-dominant—what I call a *head type*—everything is about thinking and seeing. You gauge life by reason alone, by how quick-witted and clever you are. You say to yourself, "I think you will disappoint me; love is overrated; you are only trying to manipulate me into doing something I will regret later; I'm so smart I can do whatever I want."

Some head types are so suspicious of the intentions of others that they retreat to a life where reading is more satisfying than actual human relationships. They are frozen in reaction to emotional invasion during childhood. Others are quite gregarious in the world of ideas but are detached from their feelings and sensations.

Perhaps you're not a head type, but you know one. Have you ever felt frustrated because you were held at arm's length by a friend who wouldn't express his or her feelings, or distanced by someone's ultra-logical, Mr. Spock–like behavior? You wanted to yell, "Hold me, feel me, touch me!" You admired their intricate minds and their quick grasp of ideas, but felt invalidated by their rationality and ability to coldly appraise every situation.

People who are ruled by their thoughts can become lost in their own universe designed to soothe their fear of invasion. They are caught in the ironic position of trying to stay in control by using cold, clear reason or idealized fantasy to obliterate caring. Head types can literally walk away and never look back. That's because they have discovered that emotional and physical detachment are the most powerful ways to prevent feelings of pain, loss, and fear.

When we are caught in the trap of mind over matter, we often feel exceptional and smart, much superior to those who get caught in the murky, weak, unpleasant world of emotion. Our ability to feel and accurately sense gets eclipsed by mental intelligence that has turned neurotic. We can't see how our thinking has become a defense mechanism against feeling the pain that heartbreak can bring. We need a fair witness to help us investigate how we habitually use neurotic thinking to stay detached. We need to get interested in how this detachment keeps us from living in the world of the body, from having equitable and satisfying relationships.

Do you remember Sarah in Chapter One, the woman who kept having gallstone symptoms even after she had her gallbladder removed? Her story is a great example of how a chronically fearful mind has the power to make real physical problems in the body worse, or even to cause them to appear from out of nowhere. Sarah was preoccupied with disaster scenarios, and that was what she got. Lucy's story, which follows, illustrates another defense created by a fearful mind to protect wounded instinct—absolute happiness—and how, paradoxically, it can cut off the enjoyment of sensation.

Lucy's Story:
The Negative Power of Positive Thinking

When Lucy asked to work with me, she told me she felt just fine about herself. She didn't have a problem, she just wanted to feel even better. The idea of somatics intrigued her. A student of the New Age movement, she reveled in her quick, intelligent mind and lusted after all the latest theories about the meaning of life. At twenty-eight, the world was her playground.

Tall, thin, and electric, she looked like Peter Pan. Her eyes gleamed with mischief and intelligence. Her mouth was set in a permanent smile. She was magnetic and mercurial—definitely not shy! She spoke quickly and cheerfully, and used her hands and eyes expressively.

Lucy saw herself as super-sensual, very liberal, very open, and very happy. She began the session by describing how people of both sexes were irresistibly attracted to her. "Everybody wants to sleep with me," she bragged. Fascinated by both men and women, she had enjoyed many lovers. She thought that was great and had nothing but good things to report about her sex life. "My body works great. I like the way I look. I know I can do anything I want to. I am happy as a lark."

When I asked her to tell me about her childhood, her response was short: "It was fine." Immediately, she shifted back to telling impressive stories about her present-day life and her exciting plans for the future. Lucy's style was frenetically newsy, superficial, and flat. In the middle of telling me about her plans to travel in South America, she suddenly changed the subject and asked if I could advise her on whether she should go alone or take her lover, who, she said, was pleading to accompany her. This caught my interest because it was a way to get more personal. I asked, "Is that why you're here? To get my advice about who to travel with?"

"No," she answered, with a glimmer of a frown playing across her impish face. "I think I'm here because I don't understand why it is so difficult for me to stay in a relationship. I'm always leaving. I don't want to hurt anyone, but something in me always makes me fly away. I used to think they were all pretending to be sad when I left, but lately I wonder why I don't feel anything but the desire to move on."

"Okay," I said, "if you want to understand your own motivation you need to get in your body."

The first step was to introduce Lucy to the experience of shifting her attention from thinking to sensation. I talked her through this simple relaxation exercise (you can try it too).

Try This Now:

> Sit comfortably in a chair, and take a moment to settle before you begin.
>
> When you're ready, close your eyes.
>
> Feel the weight of your body as you're sitting in the chair.
>
> Feel your back against the chair, your buttocks on the pillow, your feet on the floor, your hands in your lap.
>
> Feel the space around you. Your car in the driveway. The path to the door.
>
> Take in a deep breath through your nose and let it all out through your mouth with a audible sigh.
>
> Relax your eyes.
>
> Place one hand on your chest, the other on your belly.
>
> Feel the movement of breath in your body.
>
> Feel your heart beating,
>
> Feel the warmth of your own biology generating life.
>
> Now let your eyes come open.
>
> See the space around you as you feel your body breathing softly underneath your eyes.
>
> What is foreground for you now?

After this, Lucy became more receptive. I noticed that her face was softer, her voice lower. She was leaning back in her chair and looking at me directly. She seemed much more "in" her body. I said, "Now, tell me the story of your childhood from this place, from the voice of your body. If you can, tell me what really happened."

"I can hardly remember my childhood," she said slowly. I encouraged her to take her time. "I never had a room of my own. I had to share a bed with my mother." She paused listening to her own words and then let out a sad sigh. "I hated that. She was so invasive and needy. You know, I think that most of the time growing up my body felt numb. I mean, thank God I taught myself to read when I was three. I spent many a day buried in a book. I could imagine it all in living color, especially fairy tales and science fiction. Later on, I got hooked on erotic stories. It was like I was there. Sex between the pages of a book was far more exciting than having sex in real life." She was off to the races again—her voice high and fast as she made her story sound triumphant and exhilarating. She might have gone on and on entertaining me and avoiding the real story.

Lucy was what I call pathologically cheerful. Her optimistic outlook had become her most powerful weapon against her fear. When in doubt, just make exciting plans for the future—just act happy. "I'll eat, drink, and be merry tomorrow, even if today I die."

As she continued to look more deeply into her earliest sensate experiences, Lucy began to understand why she had used fantasy to escape from reality and how that process had worked to keep her chronically separated from bodily life. No one could affect her for very long because her mind was so much in charge. She had even trained herself to hover above her body like a camera. That way, she could avoid sensation altogether. When her eyes were open, she was in control. Her basic stance in life was, "You can do anything you want with my body but that doesn't mean you have me. You can never control my mind."

As we embarked on the process of looking at what she actually felt through her senses, a very different picture emerged. Lucy had no idea she was abandoning the realm of the body in order to avoid uncomfortable experiences that caused her to feel afraid. She had become an expert at amputating reality to fit her whim—living in her mind at the expense of her body. It was a good survival strategy.

Lucy was an only child. Her father had left when she was a baby. Her mother suffered from bipolar disorder and was unpredictable. Sometimes she would get violent and attack Lucy, accusing her of being a naughty child. The next minute she would turn around and take Lucy in her arms, telling her how beautiful and special she was. Sometimes her mother would turn her violence on herself. She had been hospitalized on several occasions for trying to take her own life. When that happened Lucy had to stay with child protective services, as there was no family to take her in. As she recalled those times, she bragged about how much the various social workers and foster parents had loved her. They never wanted her to leave and gave her lots of presents and attention.

Lucy's mother treated her more like a girlfriend than a daughter. Not only did Lucy have to sleep in the same bed with her mother, she had to listen to her chatter on about her lurid sexual fantasies. When her mother was manic, she often brought home creepy men from the bar down the street. Sometimes she'd wake Lucy and send her to the couch. Other times she'd forget and Lucy would wake up to find her mom making love with a smelly stranger. As time went on, Lucy's fantasy life grew so strong it blotted out everything. She didn't have to notice what she was feeling or who was in her bed.

When Lucy actually managed to feel sensation in my office, claustrophobic dread took over. After a number of talk and movement-awareness sessions, I asked Lucy if I could work directly on her body. She enthusiastically said yes, and jumped onto my table like a happy child. I asked her to lay on her back, close her eyes, breathe deeply, and shift her attention to the sensation of my touch on her body. It was almost impossible for her to breathe and feel sensation at the same time. Her jaw clenched, and her muscles automatically tightened when I put my hand on her belly. Touch catapulted her into a state of red alert. There was no denying that in Lucy's world, touch and danger were intertwined.

Reluctantly, she confessed that my touch felt like nails on a chalkboard. Even though she thought her mind trusted me, when I touched her body she completely freaked out. She couldn't follow my instructions to keep her attention on sensation. She'd feel sensation and then get a flashback that seemed to flood her body with fear.

It took one session a week for ten weeks for Lucy to sustain the feeling of the sensation of pleasure for the majority of a one-hour session. She had to learn how to follow her body's sensate feedback system rather than the vivid pictures that came from her childhood memories. She had to learn how to trust me as her guide.

Once Lucy experienced how past memories robbed her of pleasure in the present, she understood how poorly her mind's habit of happy, magical thinking had served her. She'd rather have her body go through the motions while her mind was ecstatic. This was why Lucy's experiences didn't stick to her. She was beginning to empathize with the pain she saw on the faces of her lovers when she merrily moved on. The truth was that she barely could remember them once she left. She was finally beginning to admit that for her, sensation and intimacy triggered fear instead of authentic pleasure.

It took more than six months of weekly meetings for Lucy to finally ask in a sad but curious voice, "How could I have believed I was enjoying everything when I wasn't even home? My heart and my body have never been hooked up. My mind dominates everything I do. If you had lived a childhood like mine, you wouldn't want to bond with anyone either. No wonder I never stay 'in' love."

For the first time in years, Lucy began to weep. Tearfully, she confessed how ambivalent she had always felt about sex. She had never had a deeply satisfying body-based orgasm. With these insights in both mind and body, Lucy was ready to begin the process of hooking her mind to her body. She literally had to reeducate herself to feel sensation, to enjoy the sensations her body was giving her, to practice staying present in her body for more than a few moments at a time.

It took another couple of months for Lucy to report she was regularly enjoying living in her body. Once she could tell her lover the truth about her fear, she was able to stay embodied during sex. That was intimacy. And this intimacy was guiding her toward feelings of healthy attachment. She heartfully invited her lover to travel with her to South America. She was enjoying the process of building a lasting relationship.

Lucy came to our last session singing the refrain from the Neil Young song "When You Dance I Can Really Love"—"I can love. I can really love. I can really love." For Lucy, acknowledging the degree of fear and control her mind had over her body and emotions was the key that allowed her to open her senses. Instead of flying frantically from one non-relationship to another, from one fantasy of life to another, she was putting down roots in the world and learning to reach out and hold on to others.

Tim's Story: Anxiety Is a Powerful Teacher

You don't have to come from a background as distressing as Lucy's to live life with the fight/flight button stuck in the "on" position. Tim's story is a good example of how the simple pressure to work hard and get ahead can overload us mentally.

Tim, a seemingly well-adjusted forty-eight-year-old television producer, came to me because he was scared. Suddenly, for no reason he could think of, he'd begun having severe panic attacks. He said it was like being possessed. Out of nowhere, he'd start to feel a tightening in his chest. Then his heart would start beating wildly. "The next thing I know, I feel like my blood is going explode out of my skin container." Scary indeed.

Tim went to the doctor, certain something awful was happening to him. But disease wasn't the problem. His blood pressure was normal, even his cholesterol levels were good. The doctor diagnosed him with panic disorder and offered medication to help control them. The doctor didn't spend much time asking Tim about his lifestyle or how he was feeling in general. The cause didn't seem to be as important as the symptoms, and whether or not they would respond well to medication. Tim wanted to get to the bottom of what was going on, so he came to me for help.

When Tim came to my office, the first question I asked was: "What do you think is the cause of your panic attacks?" He said he had no idea. His life was going very well. He had just completed a demanding project and was about to begin another. Trouble was that "these damn feelings of dread" were cramping his style, making him worry about whether he was good enough for the next job. Instead of being his usual gung-ho self, he was preoccupied with fear of failure —he was becoming the master of the worst-case scenario.

I asked him if he was sleeping well. He said he only needed to sleep about five hours a night, that he was restless and often awoke in the night thinking about what he had to do the next day. I asked him what kind of regular exercise he practiced. He said he used to jog four miles every morning and had since his twenties, but for the last couple of years he just couldn't find the time, even though he considered himself to be very disciplined. I asked him what his eating habits were like. He said he ate on the run. He was divorcing his wife of twenty years and grabbed food whenever he could. He often had "night breakfast," his name for a dinner of cereal.

I asked him what was missing from his life. He said, "I want to feel comfortable in my own skin again. These attacks make me so jumpy and moody. They muddle my mind and take away my confidence."

"What if this peace of mind you say you are looking for is contingent on changing your lifestyle in significant ways?" I asked. "The work of transformation requires perseverance and hard work. It is much more demanding than taking a pill." I went on to say that since he'd already done the work of whipping himself into a state of panic, why not take the medication and work with me at the same time. "The medication can assist you in the process of learning to take life in the body seriously. Somatic work can help to prepare you for life after medication. Are you willing to get out of the fast lane? Are you willing to take an honest look at yourself, at your habit of practicing mind over matter?" Tim answered immediately. "Yes. I'll do anything to feel like myself again."

Tim had the classic Posture of the Overachiever you tried on in Chapter Three. This is the typical Type A body posture—perfect for maintaining a high-stakes lifestyle. It is also a perfect way to create a breeding ground for ailments like chronic fatigue, panic disorder, or just plain burnout. Overachievers like Tim have no internal life. They have little respect for the natural limitations of the body. Getting the job done is most important, and that requires complete attention to work—to the outside world's competitive marketplace. Relaxation is not easily cultivated by overachievers. It can even feel threatening.

As our sessions continued, Tim began to learn how to take long, deep breaths and let them out fully. He was a linear thinker, so I asked him to practice using his senses without using language to analyze his experience. I sent him on a one-hour walk in nature and gave him an assignment: Spend fifteen minutes seeing without naming, fifteen minutes hearing without naming, fifteen minutes sensing without naming, and fifteen minutes just being. "That means giving up having to get somewhere," I told him. "Your goal now is to get to know your body's feedback system intimately, breathing deeply the whole way, allowing your body to be your guide. The answer," I added with a smile, "is blowing in the wind." Tim laughed out loud. A child of the sixties, he knew exactly what I meant.

"Don't tell me that this might turn out to be a pleasurable excursion," he said. "I thought you were going to make me feel guilty about how selfish I've been. You were going to make me go and apologize to my wife and kids about the time I spend at work instead of with them. You were going to make me admit it was all my fault."

"This is your life," I responded. "Listen to how you torture yourself. Here's the first clue to how you create your panic attacks. It might be more challenging than you think to lose your mind and begin the work of being present." Tim blushed. He had been caught red-handed. As he went off to do his assignment, I could tell he was interested.

There was nothing wrong with Tim that a little self-observation wouldn't cure. He was your basically healthy but sensorially shutdown American success story. After years of meeting deadlines and working overtime, he had forgotten how to stop the stressful merry-go-round he had chosen to ride so long ago. Tim had lost touch with the simple things in life. He was now an expert at the unnatural posture of fearful mind.

Working with Your Body to Open Your Mind

People who live life with the mind in charge, who use mind over matter to explain the way things are, can end up with the fight/flight reflex perpetually on. The habit of organizing attention around ideas that are essentially designed to protect us from danger by explaining rather than experiencing creates an over-adrenalized environment that makes it difficult to feel pleasure. The task is to learn how to trust the body and turn the fight/flight reflex off. This happens when you learn to question the fear that originates in the mind, and to experience sensation as an intelligent language. This triggers instinctive responsiveness and allows the body to respond appropriately, without premeditation.

The primary muscle blocks in a person who holds on to fear are in the eyes, forehead, and joints in general. Shallow breathing and tight muscles help to sustain an emotional climate of fear and mistrust. If you recognize yourself in the paragraph above, or in Lucy's or Tim's or Sarah's story, you might work with your body in the following ways:

1. Relax your eyes.

People who are ruled by their heads tend to have fast-moving eyes that are always busy looking around. This can engender headaches and eyestrain and a general feeling of living just above the neck.

Try this for five minutes three or four times each day:

> Sit in a safe spot and relax your eyes, face and jaw as you drop down into yourself.
>
> When you feel centered, close your eyes.
>
> Move them slowly in their sockets for about thirty seconds as you breathe deeply.
>
> Then rest your eyes and summon your fair witness.
>
> Reach down and change the channel from thinking to sensing.
>
> You can even place the palms of your hands over your eyes, cueing them to just rest.
>
> Feel the heat generated by your hands.

> Allow this warmth and relaxation to spill down into
> the rest of your body.
>
> Keep breathing fully as you bathe in this self-imposed
> environment of relaxation for as long as you can.
>
> Open your eyes and simply see.
>
> Take a few moments and then return to business as
> usual.

2. Drop into your senses.

People who are ruled by their head often stay there thinking,
with little awareness of the actual sights and sounds and smells and
feelings in their environment.

Try this as often as you can:

> Let in the scent, sound, and feel of the world around
> you.
>
> Let yourself be heavy.
>
> Leaning against a large tree or a building during a
> work break can be a wonderful way to drop into
> your senses and out of your mind.
>
> Let the scents of nature, or the world around you, fill
> your skull container.
>
> Let the breath of life fill your chest cavity.
>
> Let the warmth from your eyes move down to fill your
> belly bowl.
>
> Let bird song fill your heart.
>
> Three-dimensional living is really worth a try.

3. Open your joints

People who are ruled by their heads tend to move stiffly, without giving thought to their body's natural articulation.

Try this fifteen minutes a day:

Lie down face up on a rug or a padded mat and take in a few complete breaths.

Bring your attention to sensation and as you do, open your joints with slow, gentle movements.

Let yourself experience every joint in your body: fingers, wrists, elbows shoulders, toes, ankles, knees, hips, spine, neck . . . .

Explore how each joint moves.

Can you feel how your knee is engineered differently from your ankle?

Your vertebral joints from your hip sockets?

Your finger joints from your elbows?

Move as if you were swimming underwater.

Let the space around you be supportive, the way water is supportive.

Let yourself undulate in spiral stretches, like a snake.

Remember: Your body is not a machine that was invented in the industrial revolution.

When you are done, stand up as if you are standing for the first time in your life.

Notice the sensation of bringing your body to a standing position.

Walk around a bit and notice if your body feels any different.

When you go back to work, try to stay connected to your body.

Try to keep your joints and muscles relaxed and open.

Notice if this kind of relaxation helps clear your mind and sharpen your focus.

4. Develop a sense of your back.

People who are ruled by their minds often feel as if they are all front. Few of them have the sense that the back of their body even exists. You can lean against a wall as you do this exercise. The intention is to feel the back of yourself—to know that you are supported, not just by your intelligent mind but also by your intelligent body.

> Your body is a container.
>
> That means it has a front, a back, sides, a top and a bottom.
>
> Begin this exercise by bringing your attention to your eyes.
>
> Let your vision turn inward so that you can see into your body.
>
> Let your eyes relax.
>
> Feel how your spine is housed inside of your container, how it also has a back, front, top, and bottom and is surrounded by muscles and bones.
>
> Breathe deeply into your back two or three times.
>
> Your chest is not the only thing that expands as you breathe.
>
> Can you feel how your back expands too?
>
> Now, walk away from the wall.
>
> Lean back into yourself as you walk and try to maintain a sense of your back.
>
> Feel your feet underneath you, the foundation of the spine, as you move through space.
>
> Your eyes are soft now.
>
> You don't have to rely on them alone to tell you where and how you are.

5. Get some bodywork from a trained professional.

Many different styles of bodywork are offered these days. The most important thing is to have a good connection with the practitioner. Interview your bodyworker to make sure he or she has a lot of experience and is willing to guide you in the process of learning to choose sensation over thought. Many are adept at more than one style and will suggest what they perceive is the best method for you. Be sure to listen to them with both mind and body to determine if you are well matched. If you don't trust them from the get-go, having an embodied experience will be just about impossible.

Many head types don't have much experience with bodywork because the idea of touch is both foreign and threatening. If you feel this way, be sure to tell your bodyworker and ask how he or she proceeds with beginners. Many massage and bodywork centers also offer a hot tub or sauna before the hands-on session. This is relaxing, lessens anxiety, and might be a great way to prepare yourself for bodywork. If you feel uncomfortable taking your clothes off, know that many bodywork systems will allow you to keep your clothes on.

As you receive your bodywork session, keep bringing your attention back to sensation as you breathe deeply and fully. Try not to engage the bodyworker in conversation—that's a way of putting your mind in charge. Give yourself permission to stop the session if you feel frightened or uncomfortable. Most body therapists will understand and help to guide you into an embodied state.

6. Listen to your body's messages.

Whichever exercise you do to keep in shape, do it with your attention focused on sensation rather than on outcome. Listen to your body as if it were an ally rather than a stupid mule. Sometimes that might mean quitting early, and sometimes it might mean going a little farther.

Because we live in a culture that preaches "no pain no gain" it might be hard for you to distinguish the difference between pushing yourself to the edge and abusing yourself. If you are mind-dominant —an expert at driving your life with your mind—it is easy for you to ignore pain. You probably like to exercise with earphones blasting a lecture or book into your mind. Not a good idea. Take those earphones off and listen to the sensations your body is sending you.

Remember: There is good pain and bad pain. Bad pain comes in a spectrum: It may feel like a weird electrical twinge in your back, something that makes you suddenly go ouch, or a movement that makes you feel like you might break something. Good pain feels challenging and even exhilarating. It tells you that you are working but doesn't inhibit your movement or make you want to stop. As you learn to respect your body, you will easily recognize the difference between good pain and bad pain.

Pleasure Works! Tim's Story Continued

Tim took my instructions to heart. The walk in nature sold him on the process. He said he felt more alive after that hour than he had in years.

"It didn't hurt at all," he bragged. "I had a wonderful time with myself. Nature is so profound. How could I have waited this long to simply relax? How could I have gotten this far away from my senses when they were with me all the time?"

It didn't take long for Tim to feel lasting results. He was inspired to start jogging again, to transfer the awareness process of sensing without naming to his running regimen. He started sleeping seven hours a night and eating more consciously. He said he was beginning to have better dialogues with his ex-wife without even trying because he felt more willing to see things from her perspective. There was light at the end of the tunnel! For the first time in years, Tim was feeling spacious inside of himself. He now knew he could breathe almost as deeply sitting in front of his computer as he could while walking in a forest.

CHAPTER 9

Opening the Heart

It is with the heart that one sees rightly; what is essential is invisible to the eye.

—ANTOINE DE SAINT-EXUPÉRY,
THE LITTLE PRINCE

Feelings are powerful.

Have you ever felt hurt by the actions of a friend or loved one? They said what they said, or did what they did, and without warning you started gulping for breath as tears began streaming from your eyes. You were suddenly awash with feeling. You could no longer see or hear or reason. You could only run out of the room or collapse into a heap as your body lurched and sputtered out tears and sobs. Your feeling self was sure you were being abandoned. Your feeling self thought this person was betraying you for no reason, that they could never understand the real you—but that was not the case. Your friend stayed and tried to calm you down. Nevertheless, shortly after she left you still felt upset and foggy. Your mind couldn't turn off your feelings.

Have you ever wanted something so badly you pushed and pushed yourself until you got it and then—with hardly a blink of an eye—went looking for an even bigger challenge? Something inside just wouldn't let you stop and enjoy your victory. You couldn't rest. You couldn't take in your success. All you could do was keep on going toward winning another prize. You had your sights set on being the best, the richest, the best looking, the most powerful. That was all you were able to care about. Never mind that the others in your life were complaining that you weren't spending enough time with them, that they couldn't get your attention, that they felt like you didn't care. You were a prisoner disguised as a hero. You were addicted to winning.

Have you ever wanted something so badly you bought it even though you knew you couldn't afford it and didn't really need it? When you got it home you felt great for a day or two until you saw something else when you were out shopping. Your greedy heart convinced your more rational mind you would wither and die without this most desired object. Your needy heart took over again. Your rising credit card debt couldn't detour your compulsive behavior, that powerful feeling of wanting. The hungry ghost inside you demanded to be fed even though it could never be satisfied.

Maybe you have felt the same insatiability toward friends or lovers or food. "Feed me. Feed me. Feed me, now," your insides cried. Over time, you forced your mind and body to become slaves to your desire. Every once in a while, when your inability to pay the bills sobered you for a few moments, or you noticed how you didn't really need all of the things you just *had* to have along the way, you asked yourself, "Why?" When no answer came back, you realized you were the lonely victim of your own emptiness. You suffered with that realization for a few hours, and then you went back out to shop.

If you identify in some way with these scenarios, you have put your feelings—that is, your heart—in charge of your body. The reason these are such unsettling experiences is because your mind and body can't get a word in edgewise. They are trying to get your attention but you no longer know how to listen.

When the Bonding Response Is Broken

As you learned in Chapter Eight, it is just about impossible to feel fear and sensate pleasure at the same time. That is because each response is governed by its own distinct system. The sympathetic nervous system regulates the fight/flight instinct. The pituitary gland acts on the cortex of the adrenal gland, causing it to secrete cortisone during an emergency situation. When this happens, the parasympathetic nervous system—the system that keys the pleasure response —shuts down.

It's a brilliant design. Fear overrules pleasure in order for us to survive. But we were not designed to live in constant fear. In order to thrive and prosper, we require large doses of sensate pleasure (such as plenty of loving touch through caressing, holding, and cuddling), at least eight hours of delicious sleep every night, and regular time engaging with nature.

The bonding response is instinctive, a natural outcome of loving-kindness. It is stimulated and sustained by the direct experience of pleasure and is transmitted through such relationships as parenting, friendship, and sexuality. The bonding response is the antidote for separation anxiety and the catalyst for meaningful feelings.

To be bonded is to care. To be bonded is to belong. To be bonded is to be interdependent. When I am bonded through pleasure it is much more difficult to willfully cause harm. When I feel bonded in a healthy way, I naturally want to be of service, to make a difference, to be a good friend. I have clear beliefs that I am willing to fight for in a strong and passionate way. I want to be in relationship.

Numerous studies have shown that infants who experience the fight/flight response at regular intervals (say, in reaction to abuse, abandonment, or other ongoing parental dysfunction) find it much harder to relax even when they are safe. The same is true for these infants when they grow up, and for adults whose hectic lifestyle keeps them under constant stress. When our fight/flight instinct is stuck in the "on" position, we cannot relax easily or stay relaxed for sustained periods of time, even when we're on vacation. This can cause us to suffer from insomnia, panic attacks, and all sorts of other symptoms caused by ongoing stress.

Why are we talking about stress again? Wasn't that the problem of the head types? Well, some have speculated that one of the primary causes of stress is chronic touch deprivation. In *Touching*, Ashley Montagu writes that stimulation of the skin is essential in causing the pituitary gland to secrete the hormone prolactin, which plays an important role for new mothers in nursing their babies.

Mothers who are deprived of touch and safety during pregnancy have a diminished nurturing instinct. They tend not to hold their babies much, and are more inclined to let them cry for longer periods than other moms.

As we have seen, head-centered types react to long-term over-adrenalization by retreating to the world of ideas. Heart-centered types, on the other hand, get trapped in the realm of emotions. They literally live to feel loved, to be in relationships. They are run by their feelings.

When the Bleeding Heart Is in Charge: Holding on to Emotion

Emotion is the expression of feeling, the river that connects the ocean to the shore. We need emotion to feel alive, to feel a part of existence. Feeling compels us to reach out. When our natural instinct to bond is arrested or abused, we feel starved for body-to-body contact, for 3D love. This starvation distorts our natural hunger for physicality and pushes us out of balance. We mistakenly learn to use exaggerated emotionality to get the soul food we are unconsciously seeking. We throw tantrums, or dramatically withdraw to suffer alone, or become charming people-pleasers with little sense of self underneath.

For the heart types, everything is about getting approval. Life is gauged by "how I feel"—and "how I feel" relates to "how much I perceive you love me." Some people become perpetual hysterics, reacting to emotional neglect. Others get stuck in one feeling, like sadness, and suppress others, like joy and well-being. Have you ever felt you were being held hostage by a friend's tears, or bullied by someone's hysterical anger? Have you ever felt irritated as opposed to sympathetic when someone started crying as he told his sad story? You wanted to say, "Get over it!" because you felt manipulated by his emotionality. Unhealthy emotionality dominated the exchange. He was lost in his own melodrama, blind to the irony that when we try to force another to care about us, we run the risk of pushing them away even more.

When we are caught in the trap of seeing solely through the veil of emotion, we often feel rejected and misunderstood. Our ability to think and sense clearly and accurately gets eclipsed by our feelings of deprivation, our need for love. We need our fair witness to help us get clarity about the situation, to help us take responsibility for our own-out-of control behavior so we can have equitable and satisfying relationships.

People who rely too heavily on emotional expression limit their ability to use the other centers of perception naturally. For example, if the only way to get love and approval from Dad is to win the race, I let my desperate need for approval drive my body onward. So what if my body hurts? The feeling of getting love for winning is worth the pain. I will bop till I drop. I will make myself into the person he can love. I will fake it to make it. That can be especially true in sex. A satisfying orgasm requires both relaxed aliveness in the muscles and a clear, uncluttered mind. When I am more concerned with getting love from someone, I can't respond naturally to the messages that my body is sending. I can't be fully present.

Failing to recognize the difference between hysteria/depression and authentic emotion, between driving the mind and body with the will of emotional need rather than with the wisdom of natural intelligence, feeds the high-stress lifestyle and leaves us ultimately frustrated, inconsistent, and in unsatisfactory relationships. William's story shows how touch deprivation can affect emotional climate and influence how we develop in the body.

William's Story:
An Active Exploration of Presence

William was a comely young man from a wealthy and educated family. At first glance, he seemed to have it all. At twenty-five he had already traveled much of the world on his own and experimented with sex, drugs, and a variety of philosophies. Still, he had the nagging feeling that something essential was missing from life.

On his search to find out what it was, he took my class in somatics. After just one session, he discovered he wasn't feeling much in the realm of sensation. He was amazed—this was completely contrary to his idea of himself. He found, to his surprise, that he was preoccupied with feelings of self-pity and the nature of emotional suffering. He was drawn to people from the wrong side of the tracks, to the tragic side of life. For William, life was a veil of tears. Unlike Lucy, who forced herself to be happy, happy, happy, he wouldn't be seduced by cheerful hopes and dreams—he was positive his cup was half-empty.

William's impressive upper-class education had not prepared him to deal with the messages his body had been sending him. As a child he had suffered from severe asthma. His parents were always on guard, ready to rush him to the emergency room—and for good reason. William had almost died on numerous occasions. His condition seemed so delicate his mother was afraid to hold him. She ministered to his immediate needs but kept her distance physically. She feared touching her son might cause another attack. As a child William interpreted her behavior to mean he was repulsive and defective—he began to think of himself as too sickly to love, and envied children who got to run and swim, to wrestle and play sports.

Poor William. His asthmatic body forced him to stay at home. Cats, flowers, grassy fields, and exercise were all his enemies. He took refuge in reading books about faraway exotic worlds, where he could let his spirit bathe in feelings of freedom and bliss. Highly intelligent, William excelled academically and his teachers showered him with praise. That was nice, but for William it was the booby prize. Nothing could fix the fact that his body was defective. He felt he had been dealt a bad hand. "Why me?" he asked himself over and over. "Why me?" He grew to hate his body and didn't notice his own considerable gifts.

At puberty, William's asthma mysteriously disappeared. To everyone's delighted surprise, he grew strong and tall and stunningly handsome. Against his doctors' and his parents' wishes, he joined a soccer team. The feeling of running free fed his spirit so much he hardly noticed the pain it caused his body. After all, he was used to ignoring pain. For the first couple of years, William excelled. He was a courageous player. But he kept injuring his ankles. His legs ached all the time, his hips were tight, and he often tripped over his own two aching feet. Finally, after many injuries, the coach made William take a six-month break.

William felt as if he'd been handed a death sentence. He over-reacted, sinking into a deep depression and withdrawing from friends and family. Feeling sorry for himself, he reminded himself daily he was cursed with a body that brought nothing but pain and suffering, a defective body that kept him from his heart's desire. When a concerned friend recommended he study somatics, William decided to sign up.

In the first class, I introduced the concept of finding mental, emotional, and physical center with the following exercise, the Centering Stance (you can try it too):

Try This Now:

> Stand with one foot back and one foot forward.
>
> The foot in front should point straight ahead.
>
> The middle of the arch of the back foot should be in line with the heel of the front foot, and slightly turned out.
>
> Keep your knees soft—slightly bent, not locked.
>
> Hips, chest and face are facing front, just behind and in the direction of the front foot.
>
> Your body should feel relaxed and strong at the same time.
>
> Your mind should be alert, with breathing steady and eyes soft.
>
> At the same time let yourself feel heavy from the waist down into the legs.
>
> Lift your spine from the waist up, feeling lots of space between your vertebrae.
>
> Let the weight of gravity come down through your body into the earth.

If someone came over, put their hand on your chest,
and pushed moderately, you could stay rooted in
one place without too much effort, and without
pushing back.

You would feel your spine as the center of your body.

You would feel three-dimensional to yourself.

William was having a hard time. He couldn't hold his ground
when a much smaller and older women in the class pushed on him.
With a worried look and a dramatic wave of his arm, he called me
over for guidance. "I can't do it." he declared with a scowl. When I
tried to show him how to center himself with gravity we were both
amazed at how unsteady he was both physically and emotionally.
This big, strong young man was close to tears. He couldn't get connected to the ground and was starting to withdraw. Then I saw his
poor orphaned flat feet. He had no arch support. He was a pushover
because he wasn't grounded.

We'll never know if William's flat feet were congenital or if they
were the consequence of his sickly, sedentary childhood. Whatever
the cause, the muscles of his feet were undeveloped; his arches were
not doing their job. William literally couldn't stay balanced while
standing. No wonder he kept spraining his ankles. I referred him to
a podiatrist who fitted him for arch supports. That made a world of
difference. But there was more to the story.

When I put my hand on William's chest to test his sense of center, he half pushed back defiantly and half just stood there, resigned
to not having what it takes. This was a confusing mixed message and
I wondered why. It was as if he was all front, a handsome, stand-up,
cardboard image. He had no back to lean against and had forgotten
how to use his peripheral vision. At first he didn't notice what I was
talking about. He said that the exercise was interesting, that he was
learning a lot. Later, when he told me his story, I understood.

William was pretending to be healthy. Even though he was a
healthy, strong, and capable young man, he still thought of himself
as sickly. He hid his shame by looking good on the outside, by ex-

celling at most everything, by pushing his body to the limit. However, he usually collapsed somewhere near the finish line. Underneath his winning smile, William was disgusted by his own body. His heart and mind blamed his weak, defective body for always hurting, for holding him back. At the same time, he had no clue about how abusive he was being. He had no idea of what a normal body was capable of enduring.

We worked together to understand what had caused this estrangement, retrieving the pieces of the puzzle that had been lost during his traumatic childhood. As he learned through movement exercises, observed by his fair witness, how to adjust to his flat feet and re-inhabit his body in general, William found out how to actively participate in his own healing process. He was learning to tell the difference between his unrelenting feelings of defectiveness and simple sensation.

What a great sense of discernment to have at the age of twenty-five! As the class studied the techniques of therapeutic touch, William's transformation was palpable. He reported he could feel his body opening when someone touched him, and at the same time he could feel his heart shutting down. "How could I be fine and feel unhappy at the same time?" he wondered. This good question led him to a truth about himself that he had been avoiding. William realized that his narcissistic imagination was responsible for his belief that people only knew how defective he was, they would leave him in a second. And besides, he wanted love, not pity. Always in the midst of some tragic melodrama, he saw how the contradictions within himself were responsible for making him feel so unhappy. Perhaps the others in his life really did care for him. William was finally putting it all together.

The asthma that had kept him in a constant state of emergency, combined with his parents' kid-glove treatment, had left him both hungry for physical contact and wary of it. He had forced himself to stay quiet when he was really in a panic so he could eke out enough oxygen. Keeping still also made the invasive medical procedures less scary and painful. This had set the stage for the painful sense of estrangement that was his unrelenting companion. Even though he knew that his parents loved him very much, that the doctors were on his side, he felt sad and lonely almost all of the time. His body and soul craved to be lovingly touched and held. His neurotic mind was sure this would never happen.

He began to understand that comfort is hard to come by when the ability to distinguish between inapt touch and loving touch is overruled by feelings of loss and longing, by thoughts of self-loathing. Even though he was now healthy and blessed in many ways, he could not shake his negativity, or let anyone get close. His illness had caused him to substitute feelings for sensation, and fantasy for reality. In fact, actual physical experience, be it pain or pleasure, had very little to do with anything in his world. This had caused him to injure himself when he played sports, to foolishly push himself beyond his limits, to check out in a crisis, and to avoid contact with others.

William's present-day experience was usurped regularly by his painful past. For the most part, simple sensation triggered unpleasant memories of pain and fear, which he proudly embellished with dramatic emotional moodiness. He knew how to suffer better than he knew how to enjoy himself. To his credit, William saw how the feelings of sadness, shame, and envy had come to dominate both the mental and physical dimensions of his life—how the corporeal world eluded him. He had to be willing to break his childhood habit of feeling defective and then pushing people away.

The class taught him how to consciously experience the sensate glue of the erotic, that feeling of bonding that sticks to our bones when we have a love experience through pleasure. This was a metaphor for life in general. The moment William chose sensation over egocentric emotionality, his world shifted. He decided to drop Charlie Brown's Posture of Depression, (which you tried on in Chapter Three) and looked up and out to see the beautiful day before him. William had learned how to breathe deeply into his chest and eyes. The body-work he received in class helped him realize the chronic blockage that had set into his muscles in reaction to his asthma attacks. He let go and looked terrific.

It is a great day when such a young man makes the wise decision to live in his body. I can hardly wait to see who he becomes as he flowers into manhood.

Sami's Story: The Veil of Light Is Far More Difficult to Lift than the Veil of Darkness

Sami was a genuinely warm person. She cared about everyone she met—in the moment anyway. She was a butterfly, and treated everyone she met like a special flower. They contained the nectar she craved to feed her inexhaustible desire for attention. Her feelings were everything, and she experienced them anywhere with anyone at the drop of a hat. It was a great act.

Pretty and charming, with an emotional IQ that registered off the charts, Sami was irresistible. She knew how to get what she wanted and was on a never-ending hunt for opportunities to employ her feminine wiles and secure her inflated self-image. She connected by saying all the right things, by looking good, by unabashedly displaying feelings of love and happiness. She was the perfect example of the Posture of Emotional Self-Indulgence described in Chapter Three. She existed from the waist up, inflating her chest with inhalations that kept her primed for socializing and spending money she didn't have. Sami had shiny armor.

Behind her lovely gray-green eyes, however, Sami felt empty. At her core she was insecure, needy, and unable to bond for any length of time because there was no one home inside. She might have seemed free and spontaneous, but her deep, dark secret was that the opinions of others controlled her every move.

Early on, the best way she had found to escape herself was to become a master of disguise and intrigue, a person who could walk up to anyone and become their friend. She could change her look and her belief system to suit any occasion. She was always reading for the part of the heroine, the beautiful seductress, the most popular person. She could cry on command. She could get angry. Sami knew all the ways to win your heart. As a child she had practiced looking sexy in front of the mirror for hours at a time. She was enthralled by her own beauty and derived great pleasure from the many compliments that came her way. She felt entitled to have a life that looked as good as she did.

The problem was that as she grew older her game wore thin. Men found her enchanting until her unpredictable dramatic outbursts drove them away. She would rebel against the part she had distorted herself to play by angrily accusing her love object of imprisoning her precious spirit, of stealing her freedom by expecting her to be what she pretended. She accused them of not giving her what she really wanted. She was like Norma Jean playing Marilyn Monroe: mesmerizing on the outside, nonexistent underneath.

Sami was always on the go. She had little time for self-reflection, sleep, or just plain down time. She was never alone. She was usually in multiple relationships, moving between loves, projects, and parties—giving her heart away too fast in order to get that treasured approval. She couldn't see her perplexing contradictions, her own weird combination of entitlement and guilt. It was not surprising she spent so little time alone.

I met her when she came to study the bodywork part of my somatic training. She thought this could be her next profession. "I want to be a healer," she declared proudly. "I know I have what it takes to help people be happy. I want to have meaningful work," she said, flashing her alluring smile just long enough to turn on my red-alert button. She made me feel very nervous. I could see that this seductive woman suffered from the old giving-to-get routine, and I had to stay my impulse to bust her on the spot. I had to be willing to wait for a good opportunity to see if she might be willing to drop her act and let us know what was really going on behind the scenes.

As the wise old Sufi proverb says, "The veil of light is far more difficult to lift than the veil of darkness." Sami's act was seamless when she was socializing. She had shiny armor. It was only when she had to delve inside herself that her insecurities began to show. The exercises that asked her to shift attention to the sensations in her body as she moved in silence, eyes closed, threw her for a loop every time. After a few minutes of "trying" the exercise, she would fling her eyes open and look around. Sometimes she would end up in tears, other times she would leave in the middle to go to the bathroom—anything to escape the discomfort she felt. It was obvious that Sami didn't know what to do with herself when she wasn't the center of attention.

During the feedback portion of the class when we introduced the concept of the fair witness, Sami found the courage to share with the group the truth about her inability to concentrate, to stay present in the silence. With a chagrined look she told us how quickly her feelings took over during the exercise. "All I could do was worry about what you all thought of me. Did you like the way I moved? Do you think I'm attractive? Am I thin enough? On and on and on! My blood pressure went up just doing that exercise!"

She had everyone charmed and laughing as she went on to explain that when she imagined her classmates approved of her, she felt elated. When she imagined they disapproved, she felt awful. When the imagined disapproval got the best of her, she would open her eyes and peek. When she saw to her astonishment that no one was even checking her out—that everyone else was simply doing the exercise—it dawned on her maybe something was not quite right with her world. She began to wonder why it was so difficult for her to be alone, for her to feel her body, for her to settle down and feel comfortable inside her own beautiful skin.

I was delighted. Sami's candid questions and honest reporting about herself allowed the others in the class to get more real with her, with themselves, and with each other. We shifted from a group of individuals trying to learn a skill to a community of friends. A few people were able to tell her that even though they liked her very much, it was hard to work with her. Her palpable need for their approval got in the way. When she exchanged practice sessions, they resented all the time she took. It was difficult to relax around someone who was so "on" all the time.

"What can I do to get a handle on myself," Sami cried. "I feel so out of control." Now she was ready to begin the task of breaking her narcissistic love affair with her two-dimensional image. She was ready to face up to her own emptiness and hysteria.

By the end of the class Sami was a much more connected person. She still led with her emotions and suffered from an incessant need for attention, but less so and for shorter periods of time. She was getting bodywork to help her feel the sensate connections between her chest, pelvis, and legs. Her emotional fits were toning down because she was able to see for the first time how destructive they were. She took up the Japanese martial art aikido and started to spend regular time alone just sitting on her porch and letting her senses open.

She had given up on her narcissistic fantasy that someday, somehow, someone magical would save her from herself and provide her with the keys to the kingdom of happiness. She actually smiled and thanked me when I told her, "There are no miracle cures. It takes time and commitment to change, to develop a reliable sense of self. So please grow up that inner child of yours, graduate her, and don't bring her to class anymore. It's time for you to face the music and take some responsibility for yourself." Sami got a taste of the real nourishment that comes from being present and centered at the same time. I got the sense she was ready to sign up for the process of trading in her false self for someone real. She was on the road to becoming truly beautiful.

Working with Your Body to Open Your Heart

People who live life with the heart in charge, who use emotion without thought or sensation to explain the way things are, suffer from an out-of-balance bonding response. The habit of organizing attention around emotions that are essentially designed to get love through manipulation rather than through giving and receiving creates a hungry emotional environment that is invasive and demanding. Experience doesn't print well on watery emotion, so emotional types have blurry memory banks and standards that change with the weather. Predictably unpredictable, feeling fuels contact. The emotional types are hungry for love. They live for human contact and approval.

The task is to learn how to trust the mind and body for information about what is really going on, which happens when you learn to question your neediness and experience how thought and sensation are part of the whole. If you recognize parts of yourself in the paragraph above, or in William or Sami's story, you might work with your body in the following ways:

1. Exhale with a long, deep sigh.

If you are heart-centered, your primary muscle blocks occur across the diaphragm, in the muscles of the upper back, in the heart, and in the circulatory system. These blocks hold sensation out of the lower body, leaving you frustrated and in a state of always wanting more. You can get more centered by standing in the Centering Posture described in William's story.

When you feel grounded, try this:

> Summon your fair witness.
>
> Stand facing a wall and assume the centering posture.
>
> Extend your arms and place your palms against the wall just below eye level, fingers facing up.
>
> Your elbow should be lined up behind your wrist, your shoulder lined up behind your elbow.
>
> Push against the wall as you breathe deeply, keeping your eyes and muscles soft.
>
> Feel the weight of yourself as it distributes down into your legs and feet.
>
> Let yourself organize around your spine, your center line.
>
> Can you feel the sensation of weight in the soles of your feet?
>
> In your entire body?
>
> These are the sensations of groundedness.
>
> They become richer if you empty your mind of judgments and comparisons, if you let the sight, scent, sound, and feel of the world around you inform your experience.
>
> After a minute or two, walk around, keeping your attention focused on the sensations your body is sending.
>
> In this place called center you can feel what is called life force.
>
> You can feel the streaming of energy that gives you weight and dimension.

These feelings live deep inside.

They are the expression of sensation, the feeling that makes us feel connected and nourished.

2. Relax your muscles with slow, structured movements.

Can you tell the difference between emotion and sensation? A good way to learn is to take up a daily practice like yoga or t'ai chi. These systems introduce you to specific structured movement designed to enhance muscle and joint flexibility and strength while keeping the mind clear and the heart calm. They require discipline and concentration on sensation, on developing a sense of center. This is great for heart types, who habitually trigger intense feelings that muddle the mind and blur the senses. Patience is essential to staying calm and centered.

3. Develop a sense of emotional containment.

Emotional types tend to spill their emotions over everyone they meet. This can make other people uncomfortable, and give you a sense of being out of control. Exercise Four in Chapter Eight will help you develop a sense of your body as a container for your emotions. You can also incorporate this daily exercise into your routine:

Ground yourself every morning before you get going with your day.

Before you take the leap into feeling, remember to sense yourself three-dimensionally.

Instead of reaching out on first impulse, reach in. What if your eyes were housed in your pelvis instead of your skull? That would mean that your vision came from deep inside your body.

Drop your awareness down into your body.

Imagine that you are seeing out of your pelvis.

When seeing comes from the heartland of the body it is easier to access a true sense of center.

4. Get some bodywork from a trained professional.

Emotional types work well with structure. Choose a bodywork style that is simple and direct, geared to organizing the body around the center line, the spine. Rolfing, Alexander Technique, and Feldenkrais are good because they emphasize sensation over emotional expression. It's not that emotional expression is bad, it's just that heart types tend to lead with feeling and it is important to learn how to choose sensation over feeling at least some of the time.

The fact that wild animals rarely get hysterical tells us how dangerous and downright useless this kind of over-emotionality is. Both hysteria and depression keep us out of control. It is difficult to make a good decision when you're in a lifeboat if you're hysterical or depressed.

There's a difference between internalizing emotion and suppressing emotion. So, when you are receiving bodywork, keep bringing your attention back to sensation as you breathe deeply and fully. Give yourself permission to stop the session if you feel frightened or uncomfortable, but also try to keep your mind from switching over to the Sad Memories channel. This session should be about the practice of choosing to stay in your body, not indulging in feeling. Most body therapists will understand and help guide you into an embodied state.

5. Listen to your body's messages.

Whatever exercise you do to keep in shape, do it with your attention focused on sensation rather than on outcome. Heart types tend to use intense movement to feel rather than to sense—they would rather ignore physical pain in order to feel high. They have tons of excess energy and use aerobics to burn it off. That's fine, but it is important to remember to attend to sensation too, to listen to your body's sensations so you can quit when you are hurting. Like the head types, the heart types can push themselves over the edge, injuring themselves because they are overtired, overexcited, or overly ready. There is good pain and bad pain. When you respect your body you can recognize the difference. For more on how to recognize the difference, see Exercise Six (page 117) in Chapter Eight.

CHAPTER 10

Opening the Body

> The Baghdad of the body rises with its towers
> and gates.
> Inside it the palace of intelligence has been built.
>
> —KABIR

Anger is powerful.

Have you ever felt like you had every reason in the world to be mad at a friend or loved one but couldn't express it? They did what they did and you gritted your teeth, sucked in your gut, looked at the ground, and said nothing. You were so angry and so paralyzed—hot on the inside and passive on the outside. Nevertheless, you acted calm and collected; you were the voice of reason. Little did they know you had no other choice. Your cowed neurotic self was sure that if you expressed your anger, if you made waves of any kind, you would have to live alone forever. This person didn't mean to crash your car, or make you wait an hour, or not do what they promised—you had no right to be angry, it was your fault anyway. . . . Later, you had a dull headache and felt unmotivated and depressed as you obsessed about what you should have said to your friend. Your years of "be nice no matter what" training had worked. Your body no longer knew fully how to let its instinctive side live. You had learned too well how to turn your feelings off and keep your senses turned down low. The fact that your life's movie was being filmed in shades of gray didn't even get your dander up.

136

Or maybe you can relate to another kind of anger dysfunction. Have you ever gotten alarmingly mad at a friend for some minor transgression and flown into an uncontrollable rage with no warning? You actually picked up an object and threw it across the room, yelling and threatening do them bodily harm. You attacked your unsuspecting friend and felt justified. After you calmed down, you accused him of being hypersensitive and refused to apologize. "People shouldn't be so weak," you thought. "You should have seen what my father did to me when I screwed up!" Probably, most of your dear friends have felt forced to keep their distance after many attempts at trying to work things out. All your life you have used verbal or physical brute force to get your way. You look strong, but the truth is that you have lost your ability to be vulnerable.

Maybe the opposite is true: You've used brute force against your *own* anger when it threatens to take over. You may be a rigid perfectionist and a merciless critic while inside you are burning up. Or you may use the passive-aggressive method of stuffing anger. You hate rocking the boat, you avoid having an opinion whenever possible. You can't understand why you have no energy, why you're always late, why you just can't take action to do the things that are really important to you.

If you identify with these scenarios, you have put your repressed body in charge of your mind and forgotten how to think analytically. The reason you are so out of touch with your own need to get what you want is because your body has been muffled. It has been made dense by a lifetime of having to bridle your will, your feelings and your sense of territory.

When the Territorial Response Takes Over

The territorial response is the instinct that tells us where our boundaries begin and end. It compels us to fight for what is ours and to respect what belongs to others. Anger is the response nature gave us to enforce these boundaries. When the communication lines between mind and body are cut early on, the expression of anger either gets out of control, becomes paralyzed, or turns inward, polluting us with resentment and blame. Each distortion is driven by particular kinds of muscle armor designed to muffle both feeling and bonding.

What does healthy instinctive anger look like? Nature equipped us with the ability to get angry for good reason. It is natural to fight to protect hearth and home. It is natural for our hair to stand up on the back of our neck when someone bigger and stronger uses inappropriate anger as a weapon against someone smaller and weaker. The first is animal instinct, the second is animal instinct plus moral code. In either case, the healthy expression of anger works when it protects by doing the least amount of harm to both parties, when it gets the intruder to back off, when it passes quickly.

Have you ever approached a mother dog with her new pups? If you get too close, all she has to do is raise her upper lip and utter a low growl. A normal, well-meaning human or dog will back off without testing the situation further. Rational thinking has little place here—our gut gets the message loud and clear. So what is it that can alienate us so totally from natural impulse? How is it so many women allow their husbands to abuse them and their children? How is it so many men become bullies?

When the Repressed Body Is in Charge: Holding on to Anger

When the expression of natural instinct is forbidden with no good explanation, when the cultural mind dominates biology unconditionally, neurosis and sometimes perversion set in. Can you remember a time when you knew you were angry and had to hold your body and your tongue? How did you do it and how long did the feeling last? Did you hold your breath and tense the muscles around your lower back and pelvis? Did you force your mind to imagine something else? Did you cry instead? Did you decide to take vengeance by retreating as you feigned emotional indifference? All are sometimes understandable responses. But what if you chose this reaction for a lifetime? What if shutting down anger shuts down passion and will and creativity? What then?

People who rely too heavily on territorial imperative limit their ability to use the other centers of perception naturally. For example, if the only way to assure my privacy is to attack anyone who trespasses, I end up scaring off friends. If I let my obsessive need for tidiness override my desire for having fun, I become uptight and rigid. I let my desperate need to establish boundaries drive my heart into seclusion and keep my mind locked in black-and-white thinking. So what if I have no friends? The sense of securing control through the establishment of rules or physical boundaries is *worth* the isolation. I will be *right*. I will enforce the rules. When I am more concerned with breaking and making rules than I am with caring for others, I can't respond naturally to life. I can't be fully present.

Remember Janice, the fiercely driven, work-obsessed Silicon Valley marketing executive, from Chapter Two? She is an example of what happens when anger gets turned inward and duty overrides compassion. Her obsessive-compulsive perfectionistic approach to everything made her anger manifest as corrective resentment. She expressed it in her persnickety enforcement of the rules, by taking it on herself to be everyone's critic. George, on the other hand, was simply obsessive. His story is a good example of the price paid for the chronic repression of healthy, instinctive anger. It makes us passive-aggressive.

George's Story:
Cutting Off Your Arms to Spite Your Father

Time had turned George into a curmudgeon. This tall, pale, stoop-shouldered fifty-year-old engineer had come to one of my somatic workshops because he said he was "feeling blah." That was obvious. He passively stood aloof from others in the group, revealing practically nothing about himself. The most he would share was the memory of a mind-expanding experience he had had during the sixties. In a resigned monotone, he said he was seeking to rediscover that sense of excitement and good will he had felt then. He was the perfect model for the Posture of Depression (with a touch of the Posture of Compliance) described in Chapter Three.

After the first meditation exercise, he sarcastically shared that he had "nearly fallen asleep." Following a movement exercise, he said (with a bit more surprise and sincerity) he had enjoyed the exploration but was disturbed by the stress and pain he was now aware of in his shoulders. I shared with him my observation that his arms were hanging pendulously from his shoulders, reflecting his reported state of blah. I suggested that before the next class he pay attention to how his arms worked during regular life activity.

At the evening Gestalt group, George startled everyone when he snapped at a man who had just shared an intimate story about his relationship with his young son. When confronted, George denied his comment had sounded hostile or that he felt angry in any way. When I said, "I heard more than feedback in your voice. You sounded like you wanted to punch his lights out," he denied it. "Well." I said, "when have you felt anger in your life, and who provoked it?"

George replied without hesitation, "My father, when I was a child."

He then recounted that he was feeling very troubled by his sensate observations during his time away from class. He had noticed he had very little feeling in his arms, and for that matter, in his body in general. Even more disturbing were the memories of his childhood that were suddenly playing back like movies in his mind. He told us how he often missed catching balls, dropped things a lot, and had felt oafish, especially because his father was a successful athlete and insisted on him following in his footsteps. He was average at almost everything. He was guilty of the American sin of being just mediocre and was doomed to suffer the humiliation of his father's cruel teasing and obvious disappointment. This curse followed him into adulthood. He had internalized the critical voice of his father, regarding his body with disfavor and resentment.

George went on to reveal that when he was a boy his father frequently beat him with a strap. In a soft, flat voice he went on to say that sometimes his father would make George get the strap for his own beating and sometimes he would attack out of nowhere. George's voice got softer, and his entire demeanor shrank as he told the truth of his horrible secret history. I asked him to tell the story again and feel his arms at the same time. He did and began to tremble. He was there, regressing to the feelings of a small helpless boy in the face of danger. He said, "I always wanted to hit my father back. I was a coward."

I put a large pillow in front of him and told him to see his father on it and tell him how he felt about him. He did so quite timidly, his arms immobile at his sides. I encouraged George to use force, to lift his arms and hit the pillow. Collapsing into a tired heap he whined, "I can't. This feels so stupid. What's the point anyway? My father is dead."

"Let's not analyze it just now, George." I said. "Come on, do you want some help or are you just going to do what you usually do, give up?" I knew I was being hard on him but I wanted to get his dander up. Maybe getting mad at me would work better.

"All right, all right," he whined some more. "What do you want me to do?" Once again, I told him to call the spirit of his father into the room, to see him on the pillow, and to tell him how he felt about the way he had fathered him. "You shouldn't have hurt me like that," he said, in a barely audible voice.

"Tell him: 'Don't you ever hit me again!'" I growled. He did and his real rage broke through. George's body got big, his voice menacing as he punched his imaginary father and demanded he "Get off my back, you motherfucker! I will never let you beat me again," he said over and over again as he brought his formidable fists down hard onto the pillow.

Time stopped. We were all moved by his work and inspired by his courage. George looked great. He emerged from the session with color in his cheeks and a mischievous smile on his face. His eyes were bright, his chest was expanded, his voice was strong and clear. "Thank you" he said, "that was very satisfying."

"What are you most aware of in your body right now?" I asked.

"My arms are tingling. They feel more attached to my body. And I feel so awake, so clearminded."

I told George, "In healthy families, fathers allow their sons to experiment with their power. They are guides, not dictators. As a child, the only way for you to cope with your father's brutality was to amputate your anger. In order to do this you had to keep your arms lifeless and close to your sides. Symbolically, you amputated them to play your father's scapegoat. If you had no arms, not only couldn't you hit, but you couldn't reach out for love or help. Worse than that, you couldn't hold anyone close. You couldn't express your love."

George's territorial instinct had been arrested. He had never been allowed to mark his territory emotionally, physically, or intellectually because his father insisted on being the "alpha dog." The best defense mechanism George could find was passive-aggressive compliance. He accomplished this by holding his breath and tightening his muscles, especially around his throat and anus. This is the formula for imploding all feeling, for living in a state of tolerable depression, supported and maintained by a general body numbness. Both pleasure and pain are erased. It is like living in a well-sealed, soundproof room. Nothing can get in, and nothing can get out.

To break free of this lonely prison, George had to start moving. He had to intentionally allow himself to breathe deeply into his chest. He had to stay present and not allow the past to shut him down. I recommended he start jogging or playing tennis so that he could get his heart pounding and his blood circulating. He needed to breathe hard and sweat. He would also benefit from some kind of deep tissue massage that helped to elongate his muscles, to get the knots out. He needed help in opening his muscles and bringing the full-range sensations back to life.

George listened carefully. With eyes full of appreciation he asked me, "How do you know this? How could you hang in there with me when I got so loud and angry? My wife can't tolerate anger of any kind. I've lived in constant fear of harming her and our children. Something awful might happen if my rage got out of control."

I said I was passing on a lineage I had received from my teacher Robert Hall; a lineage he had received from his teachers and they had received from theirs. Just as George had been able to evoke the spirit of his father during the Gestalt session, I was able to evoke Robert Hall's spirit to give me courage and keep me centered. Not only that but I had the support of my long-time teaching partner, Robert Sanoff. "None of us does it alone," I said.

"We get wounded in relationship and we get healed in relationship. We teach what it is we most need to learn, and so it goes. Now that your anger is visible, you have an opportunity to learn how to use it in a healthy way, how to disarm it rather than surpass it. Congratulations on doing a brave and inspiring piece of work."

George had clearly been touched, mentally, emotionally and physically. By the end of the workshop, he enthusiastically engaged in conversation with other participants and was able to express his appreciation with a warm hug as he said good-bye to each of his new-found friends. I hope he got enough strength and insight from this short workshop to continue the rebirth of his life-force at home with his family.

Carla's Story: A Little Truth Goes a Long Way

A few years ago, I volunteered to work with women inmates at a prison not far from where I live. The medical director at the prison was interested to see if the awareness techniques employed by somatics would help relieve stress and improve communication.

Because they lived in a prison the women were up against themselves on many levels; all their power was taken away; their every move was supervised. They were told when to wake up and when to sleep, when to eat and when to wash, when to work and when to play. The only way to cope was to surrender, and that is not easy for anyone, especially for those who had spent a lifetime fighting back. Their sense of territory was violated every single minute of every single day.

Carla's story stands out as an example of what happens when rage that is usually in your face is forced underground, when your sense of dignity is undermined.

Carla was big and strong and scary—five foot nine inches and 170 pounds of hard, dense muscle. The moment I laid eyes on her I knew I was in the presence of a powerful person, someone who had lived a life where anger and vengeance were the coin of the realm, where viciously fighting back was the only way to get somewhere. She had grown up in the Detroit ghetto, the second of ten children. Early on, she learned how to take charge by being tough, brutally honest, and invulnerable. Carla fought to win, mentally, emotionally and physically. Her body language exemplified the posture of aggression described in Chapter Three.

Now she was doing twenty-five years for dealing drugs. According to her she had been trapped by circumstance. If she plea-bargained for a shorter sentence by ratting on her husband, by revealing his sources, they would come after her when she got out. Her only choice was to keep her mouth shut and do the time. But these days, doing the time was worse than death because she was doing most of it in solitary confinement.

Carla not only didn't know how to contain her anger and hostility, she had never even considered it. She radiated insubordination. Her sense of justice compelled her to stand up for who she considered to be the underdog. Needless to say, that strategy doesn't work well in prison. You can't attack a guard who you feel is abusing a fellow inmate, or a fellow inmate who you think is abusing you. You either have to ask for help from the authorities or get out of the way.

Unfortunately, a lifetime of might over right had eliminated the words "can't" and "help" from Carla's vocabulary. She was in a perpetual state of fighting back. The fact that she now had no outlet for her "alpha dog" behavior was literally making her sick. Solitary confinement was not her cup of tea. It made her feel crazy inside. She hated being alone. However, because she believed that showing weakness of any kind was unacceptable, she maintained a defiant exterior. It wasn't until she had a seizure in solitary that things started to change. Her seizures were serious. It seemed as if her anger was so imploded that her brain exploded.

I met Carla shortly after her seizures began. The prison doctor told me they had not found a physiological reason for her condition. The doctor was concerned about Carla's inability to adjust to her situation and wondered if I would show her some relaxation techniques —that is, if Carla would even be open to the somatic approach.

Carla came to a class I was teaching at the prison on the "Art and Practice of Living in Your Body." I was explaining how the body reflects the mind, how important it is to live in your body to find balance mentally, physically, and emotionally. Basically, I was explaining the contents of this book, followed by exercises and group feedback. Carla raised her hand about ten minutes into my lecture before I had shown them any of the exercises.

"I can't relate." she said. "Relaxing is dangerous in prison." She was formidable. I had to take a deep breath and hold my own ground to come up with an appropriate response. I looked her straight in the eyes and said, "Tell me more."

She said in prison if you let your guard down for a second you would lose your power, you would lose everything. It wasn't worth it. "What do you know, anyway?" she quipped. "You're just trying to relieve your middle-class guilt."

I was impressed by her honesty, dignity, and intelligence. I acknowledged her and said, "I'm not here to debate you, Carla. I'm here to offer some coping skills. You're right. We're from different worlds, and I can understand why you don't think I'm trustworthy. As far as I'm concerned you can leave. There's no rule that says you have to be here. But if you can cut me some slack and give me a chance, I'd be more than happy to work with you. If I'm on the wrong track you can tell me, but as a friend rather than an enemy. I'm not willing to be intimidated by you. If I was on your turf, I'd be wary. But right now, like it or not, you're a prisoner and I have the upper hand."

To my great surprise she broke into a smile that lit up the room. Looking at the others she said, "I like her. She's got style." Looking directly at me again she said, "All right. Tell me your deal."

I said, "Your tough attitude and your body are partners in a crime you're committing against yourself. If you want to feel better you have to stop attacking and start listening. You have to be willing to breathe deeply into your heart and body. You have to be willing to interrupt the melodrama tape in your mind that tells you a million times a day you're a victim. You have to find a way to care about yourself. I can show you how to use your breath combined with gentle stretching to begin the task of disarming your muscles. I can show you how to choose the sensation of simple pleasure over obsessive thinking. These are the first steps in the process of stress reduction, in the process of authentically forgiving those who have wronged you, especially yourself. You have all the time in the world to practice and it will take everything you have to stick to the program."

Carla roared at me. Her body got even bigger as she leaned forward and said, "You expect me to forgive those motherfuckers who ruined my life, who put me here in this hell hole, who oppress me every day? There's no way. You gotta be dreaming."

"That's it!" I said. "You're doing it right now. This is how you make your life even more unbearable. Look at you. You're all puffed up. You're ready to jump me on account of an idea you disagree with. I could call a guard and get you sent down right now. Come on, get a grip. At least talk to me like I'm a human being. I don't deserve to be treated like this. I'm not the one who landed you here." The other women nodded and cheered me on. Once again a big beautiful smile lit up her face. "You're good," she said. "Okay, show me this breath thing."

A little truth goes a long way. No one had ever taken the time to explain to her how anger works. Armed with some understanding of how the human animal is instinctively programmed, Carla could see and hear and respond with dignity and containment. She could express her power in a new way. She had some tools to go with the rules and she was interested.

Even though I could only come to the prison once a month, there were other volunteers who worked with Carla, teaching her the basics of meditation, conscious movement, and the concepts of forgiveness and surrender. Slowly but surely, Carla began to soften. She was a heartful human being underneath her menacing exterior. We had given her a way to keep her spirit strong. Now she wanted to learn how to cultivate the seeds we were planting inside her. Her seizures stopped. She hardly ever had to be sent to solitary. Carla was learning how to speak her mind while keeping her body centered.

To my great dismay, I didn't get to work with Carla for very long. Out of the blue, it seemed, she was transferred to another prison. I didn't even get to say good-bye. I think of her often and pray she has been able to continue working on herself. She helped me to see how ignorance plus maltreatment breed toxic reactionary behavior—that heartfelt education and kindness really do work.

My work at the prison changed me too. Every time I left I felt so grateful to be free. At the same time, I began to see we are all doing time in the prison of ourselves. We are all at the mercy of self-appointed mean prison guards who keep us in isolation and despair. We are all like Carla. The hard work of breaking through our narcissism is imperative in order to change. We have to take off our suit of armor before we can experience the joys of being vulnerable.

Working with the Body to Open the Body

People who live life with their repressed bodies in charge, who use matter over mind to explain the way things are, can end up with malfunctioning territorial responses. The habit of organizing attention around physical reality alone keeps them oblivious to their own needs. Some people can get caught in the inessentials of life—working too long at a job that doesn't suit them, or postponing a project that is dear to their hearts. Some become rageful bullies, lashing out to protect the weak instead of working to find a peaceful solution. Others obsess on the rules so much they become incapable of approaching anything close to creative solutions.

A body that is forced to regularly repress instinctive anger acquires a thick skin, a density that keeps the spirit narcotized against feeling emotions. Even though this type of person is primarily sensate (organizing attention around physical phenomena that occur both inside and outside the body), the absence of clear thinking and feeling dulls the capacity to be sensitive and responsive.

The head types, because of their over-reliance on thought and mental imagery, are often accused of having bad memories in regard to social interaction. Body-based types, on the other hand, say that experience prints directly onto their bones, producing indelible, three-dimensional memories. This is because they honor the power of physicality. They believe unflinchingly in the existence of solid reality and tend to be literal. They look to the past to validate the present and have consistent internal moral standards, sometimes to a fault. Extremely willful, these types are overly concerned with territory, with both the making and breaking of the rules. They can definitely hold a grudge. Their stories always include place, time, and temperature, along with a moral.

The body-based types have trouble with emotional expression in general. The body reflects this brilliantly, with dense muscle designed to keep both the bad guys and the feelings out. The task is to use the expression of authentic anger to open, and then heal the heart. Somatic practices teach that when balance is restored to the body, anger transforms into excitement, allowing spontaneity and creativity to flow.

If you recognize something of yourself in the paragraph above, or in Janice's or George's or Carla's story, you might work with your body in the following ways.

1. Open the spine.

For repressed body types, the primary muscle blocks are most often found in the muscles of the pelvic floor (especially the anal sphincter) and in the short muscles that support the spine, jaw and neck. Opening the spine is essential for conducting feelings of connection and peace.

You might try this:

> Stand with your legs shoulder distance apart, knees soft and slightly bent.
>
> Inhale as deeply as you can and let all the breath out through your mouth with a big, audible sigh.
>
> From standing, drop your chin slowly to your chest, feeling the sensations in each vertebrae of your neck.
>
> Continue bending your body over, rolling down, vertebra by vertebra.
>
> Let your head and arms hang like a rag doll as they get closer and closer to the floor.
>
> Once your torso is hanging down comfortably over your legs, stay there for a minute, relaxing and allowing your spine to open.
>
> Come up by lifting from the lower back.
>
> You are stacking your vertebrae one on top of the other from the bottom up.
>
> When you are fully standing, stretch your arms out to the side and up over your head, arching your back slightly.
>
> Lower your arms to your sides and notice the sensations you are feeling.

Repeat the exercise three times, remembering to breathe into your back as you go, putting your attention on sensation.

2. Feel what's in the container.

Try this now or when you can:

> Put on an ambient music CD
>
> Lie down on your back and close your eyes.
>
> See if you can feel the bones inside your body.
>
> Breathe into your body in a way that makes you feel the space inside the container that is you.
>
> Gently move your joints and stretch your muscles.
>
> Let yourself be light and airy.
>
> Keep your movements small and simple.
>
> Move and stretch for about ten minutes.
>
> Then stop, close your eyes, and feel the sensation in your body.
>
> Can you tell the difference between emotion, sensation, and thought?
>
> Start moving again, letting sensation be your guide.
>
> Stretch your muscles like a sensuous cat.
>
> Don't go for the burn, go for the pleasure.

3. Develop a sense of permeability.

Try this now or when you can:

> Put on a CD of waves breaking on the shore, or better yet, go to the beach.
>
> Lie down in the fetal position (on your side, knees bent comfortably).

Close your eyes and breathe deeply.

Let your skin be alive with sensation.

Can you feel your heart beating?

Can you feel your chest expand as you inhale and
  exhale?

What if you had never used your legs for walking—if
  you were underwater and could move them around
  easily?

Try it.

Let your legs twist and swim in the airy water that
  surrounds you.

Let them push against the floor that supports you.

Feel how they connect into your hip sockets, how
  your hips move your pelvis, how your pelvis moves
  your spine.

Let your legs sway like seaweed in the ocean, like tree
  branches in the wind.

Let your whole body ride in the waves of movement.

When sensation reaches the heart it is easier to access
  true feeling.

4. Get some bodywork from a trained professional.

Repressed body types respond best to deep tissue massage combined with joint manipulation. The Feldenkrais system is great for
opening the body in a way that brings better function to the joints
of the body. People with dense muscle armoring tend to hold back
at the joints, inhibiting emotional expression

When you are receiving the session, keep bringing your attention back to sensation and ask yourself, "What am I feeling?" Give
yourself permission to receive this pleasure and sometimes pain. Consider forgiving an enemy—letting yourself be open to change. This
session is about the practice of choosing to feel yourself. It is difficult

to feel when you are polluted inside by thoughts of intense resentment and blame. That's why it is essential for body-based types to cultivate the attitude of forgiveness. The relaxation and vulnerability created by bodywork helps stimulate the capacity to forgive, to get on with life in the present. Most body therapists will understand and help guide you into an embodied state. Breath work is also quite helpful in the release of anger and built-up tension.

5. Take up tennis or some sport that makes you breathe hard and break a sweat.

Play with your attention focused on your emotional state rather than on being dutiful. Listen to your heart as if it were an ally rather than a blithering fool. Let yourself have fun. Play to feel yourself rather than to win. Remember to breathe. Remember to feel all the segments of your body, let yourself be light and airy and permeable. You might do Exercise 1, "Opening the Spine," before you begin to play the sport you've chosen.

Improvisational dancing is also great for body types. Some cities have a center where you can dance improvisationally. A DJ plays a variety of music in a smokeless, alcohol-free environment. Participants can dance alone, with a partner, or even with a group. It's a place to just let your body have a good time. The goal is to be unselfconsciously connected to yourself, to feel your sensations and feelings and to have a good time.

PART THREE

With Senses
Wide Open

CHAPTER 11

Being Here Now

> When we come to a point of rest in our own being,
> we encounter a world where all things are at
> rest, and then a tree becomes a mystery, a cloud
> becomes a revelation, and each person we meet a
> cosmos whose riches we can only glimpse.
>
> — DAG HAMMARSKJÖLD

Doing the exercises in this book will give you a good start toward opening your senses in a real and physical way. It is also helpful to take up an ongoing body discipline in which sensation is the active stabilizing focus of attention—t'ai chi, yoga, or a martial art like aikido. The slow repetition of memorized movements teaches you how to stay grounded in your body and when to use sensation as a trustworthy guide. You usually need to practice the art of being centered in a safe space, on a regular schedule, and with a teacher who can help you come back to center when you get off balance.

We can be so good at our conditioned tendencies that we mistake them for balance. However, if you are reading this book, you probably suspect that you are out of balance to some degree. Moshe Feldenkrais said, "Habits are the hardest things to notice." He also articulated this important point about practice and awareness:

154

We tend to stop learning when we have mastered sufficient skills to attain our immediate objective. Thus, for instance, we improve our speech until we can make ourselves understood. But any person who wishes to speak with the clarity of an actor discovers that he must study speech for several years in order to achieve anything approaching his maximum potential. An intricate process of limiting ability accustoms [us] to make do with [a small part of our] potential.

No one is perfectly balanced. Even the masters need to practice every day. As you do the Centers Practice that follows, remember these words of Morihei Ueshiba, the man who invented aikido: "It is not that I don't get off center; I just correct so fast that no one can see me."

Centers Practice: Bringing Yourself Back Home

You can do this exercise every day, or as often as you feel necessary. The point is to bring your dominant center down to size, and to give your less dominant centers some space to expand. It works best when someone reads the exercise to you. Next best is to feel sensation in your body from the inside out as you read the words.

The Belly Center

Stand up and get into the centering stance position.

When you feel centered, close your eyes and breathe deeply into your belly.

Let all thought and worry go.

Clear your mind, summon your fair witness, and shift your attention to sensation.

I promise that all the important things you have to think about will wait while you do this exercise.

The Belly Center is located just below the diaphragm.

It includes the organs of the liver, gallbladder, large
     and small intestines, bladder, reproductive organs,
     genitals, anus, and surrounding bones, nerves, and
     muscles, as well as the legs and feet.

It also includes the skin.

Now, place the palm of one hand on your lower
     abdomen, between the naval and pubic bone.

Place the palm of the other hand on your lower back.

Feel the container of your abdomen from the inside,
     as it expands, and from the outside, with the nerve
     endings of your palms, as your lower body pushes
     into its own hands.

Your pelvis is three-dimensional.

Can you feel your genitals and anus sitting in the
     pelvic floor?

Can you feel your intestines resting between your
     lower back, or lumbar spine, and your belly?

Feel the pressure of gravity making you heavy,
     bonding your feet forever to the ground.

Feel your hip joints and upper legs extending out of
     your pelvis, your knees, lower legs, and feet as
     they connect you to the earth.

Imagine that out of each of your feet there extends a
     root-like cord that grows down into the core of the
     earth. The direction is infinitely down.

This is the place where primary instinct lives.

There is no language here.

No concerns about time or space.

No past or future.

No moral code.

Trees and rocks occupy this place.

There is nowhere to go.

No social life.

No emotions.

Only the eternal now.

Here sensation predominates.

We are free to just be.

But please, be careful. The belly center can also be a trap.

When we live here out of habit combined with no awareness, a kind of lethargy sets in.

Without the ability to feel and think, we are lost in a timeless indolence of spirit.

When you connect to this place, take your hands away and walk around.

Better yet, walk outside in nature with senses wide open, like a lion on the African plain, or a tiger in the jungle.

There are no deadlines here, just the call of instinct to guide your way.

The Heart Center

Come back inside and find the centering stance again.

As you do, shift your breath from your belly up into your chest, eyes softly closed.

The Heart Center is located mostly in the upper back and chest.

It contains the heart, lungs, diaphragm, and rib cage, the upper back, shoulders, arms, and hands.

It also includes the neck, throat, larynx, trachea, mouth, lips, teeth, and tongue.

Place your left hand over your heart and your right
hand on top of the left.

Feel your rib cage and muscles from the inside out as
they expand and contract.

This is the place where unconditional love lives.

Quan Yin, the Buddhist goddess of unbearable
compassion, resides here.

Slowly, as if you were under water, extend your arms
out from your heart into the space around you.

Feel how your fingers are connected to your hands,
are connected to your wrists, are connected to your
lower arms, are connected to your elbows, are
connected to your upper arms, are connected to
your shoulders, are connected to your chest and
upper back.

The chest cavity contains your heart and lungs in the
front, your scapula or wing bones and thoracic
vertebrae in the upper back.

This is the place of giving and receiving, the place
where the heart connects to the hands.

As you extend your arms and then return them to
your heart, imagine yourself extending and
receiving unconditional regard to and from all
sentient beings.

The direction here is infinitely horizontal in all
directions.

Emotional bonding and relationship live here.

This is where expression comes from.

But please, be careful.

When we are caught in the Heart Center, we get
needy and greedy, clingy and jealous.

We act out our emotions to get attention.

Emotion without body and mind can't feel itself.

When this happens we feel empty and others feel burdened.

When you connect to this place, take your hands away from your heart and walk around.

Better yet, walk outside in nature with senses wide open, as your arms and hands take in the sensation of the cool air.

From this place I ask you: Who do you love?

Who do you know loves you?

How do you know?

Reach out and touch something or someone from this place.

Notice what it feels like to give and receive at the same time.

There is so much, plenty enough to go around.

There is no pretending here, just pure emotion to guide you on your way.

The Head Center

Now, come back to the centering stance once again.

As you do, let your breath move up from your chest cavity, into your eyes.

Let your eyes be open and unfocused.

Let light and shadow enter without language.

The Head Center is located above the neck.

It includes the eyes, ears, skull and cognitive center of the brain.

There is no emotion here, just extreme lightness and clarity that is driven by mental acuity.

Mind at its essence is like a giant radar dish, receiving all the thoughts that have ever been thought—and some that haven't.

We are like spirit here. We have access to profound knowledge in this place. Languages, math, physics, and music are processed here.

Reach your arms up to the heavens, with hands wide open.

There is no weight or sensation to keep you on the ground, no limit to your visual imagination.

The direction here is infinitely up and out.

But please be careful.

To be stuck here, without feelings and sensations, is to be unable to love.

Without feeling and sensation it is difficult to attach to anything but two-dimensional ideas.

Understanding is not enough.

Without feeling and sensation, this becomes the place of the frozen heart.

When you connect to this place, take your hands down and walk around.

Better yet, walk outside in nature.

Take in the world around you with your sixth sense, your intuition.

The other five are not active here.

Let your thoughts and visualizations run free.

The body merges with space, leaving pure knowing to guide you on your way.

Now, come back to the centering stance one more time.

Slowly, bring yourself back to right now, to right here,
to present time.

Look around you: What do you see?

Listen: What do you hear?

Be aware of your skin: What does it feel?

Inside your mouth: What is the taste?

Inhaling: What do you smell?

Feel your centers in balance with each other.

No fighting for control, no relinquishing power.
Just being.

Now, mark this place so that you can return to it
whenever you like.

Open your eyes and come back to everyday reality.

It can be difficult to bring this peaceful state into a hectic lifestyle, so go easy on yourself. The privacy of your own home is like a
sanctuary; the crowded freeway of life is where practice doesn't always translate easily into reality. Remember to be patient as you bring
yourself back to everyday life, as you prepare yourself to go out into
your world. You might not want to do this meditation before you go
food shopping or balance your checkbook. Reserve it for when you
have the time to explore what I call "essence."

Essence

At home in our bodies, at home on the planet, we are at rest. This
gives us the wonderful opportunity to go deeper into the place of
essence that connects us to each and every being. This is a place
where we no longer worry what anyone thinks about us; a place
where we can just be. Paraphrasing Rumi, Coleman Barks says it this
way: "What may seem at first to be an emptiness of no consolations,
no desire, a grand aloneness, becomes garden-like. You walk the open-
roofed sanctuary, between the lines of trees, rabbits in the aisles."

This place of essence is elusive. It disappears when thought and
desire try to box it in, or when we project it onto others. Wise teachers

show us that we can enter this world by training our attention, by practicing exercises designed to help us let go of our conscious bias toward physical truth and awaken to the simultaneous reality of the truth of the spirit. This is not a place that denies the body, but a place that rejoices in the body's ability to contain and express the essence that is at once our unique being and connection to the universe. The following story is a great example of the role sensation plays in the process of experiencing essence.

Michael's Story

Michael, a very savvy Catholic priest, attended a somatics workshop I was teaching. A doctor of psychology, he was interested in the somatic approach. From his first words it was clear he had prepared for my workshop by studying whatever he could find written on somatic theory. He had a good sense of himself and put me on the spot, asking questions that were difficult to answer.

Out of his stiff and blocky body shone a pair of clear-seeing overused eyes. It was obvious that Michael had not used his body as a resource in a long, long time. To his credit, he understood he had chosen to abandon the realm of the body because he was convinced this was the price for living a pious life. Instead, he chose to live in the cool, dry domain of insightful thought, venturing only occasionally into the regions of sainted bliss. He had studied the teachings of Jesus and had given his life to practicing what he preached. Nevertheless, he was lonely. He knew his cool detachment made him stubborn and intimidating—it forced his colleagues to keep their distance. Was it the Catholic emphasis on mind over matter and his vows of celibacy that kept him feeling imprisoned in a body that wouldn't bend? His psychology training combined with his latest study of somatics made him suspicious that this stiff body of his might be the reflection of a closed heart. He had come to my workshop to explore this possibility.

Even though he was a body type, the centering stance exercise eluded Michael. No matter how hard he tried to burrow in, I could push him over easily. His body was seriously locked up. He wore a girdle of muscle just to keep his shoulder joints from moving separately from his chest and upper back. He made himself denser and denser by locking his joints and holding his breath. It was as if he had studied body technique with a Brahman bull! Under this kind of physical pressure, however, his habit didn't serve him and he was visibly upset. He hated not being able to control his control.

As difficult as it was for Michael to make changes in himself, he was intrigued by the transformations he saw in the other people in the group as they discovered how to center themselves. He could see that the somatic method of combining meditation, movement awareness practices, emotional release work, and telling your story from the voice of the body was a powerful catalyst for restoring balance. But no matter how hard he tried, Michael couldn't quite break out of his cerebral prison. He asked me what other techniques might help him, and I asked if I could touch him—if I could do a bodywork session on him in front of the group. Happily, he agreed.

I asked him to lie face up on a mat in the center of the circle. Everyone else was to stay present and be silent as they watched us work. I told Michael, "Please don't hesitate to stop me for any reason, at any time. This is not about enduring. It is about being." He smiled and looked at me through beautiful, intelligent eyes.

"Now close your eyes and take some long, deep breaths," I began. "Feel your back on the mat, the air on your skin, all the sensations in your body. Keep your attention on the feelings in your body as I touch you. When you find your mind trying to analyze my strategy, or remembering something from your past, or worrying about what we all think of you, simply bring yourself back to the sensations you are feeling, to your breath. Let your fair witness and my hands be your guide."

Armed with the precious tools of my own experience and training, with the empowering sensate memory of my father's healing touch on my cheek, of Randy's hands on my knee, of Robert's authentic presence, I put one hand on his breast bone, the other underneath his right shoulder. I pushed down from the top, which allowed me to rock him gently from side to side as I pushed up from underneath into the muscle between his scapula and his spine. My touch was directive but uninvasive. I wanted him to feel himself, not me. I worked slowly, leaving a lot of space between touches. I could feel Michael's attention getting deeper along with his breath. There was nothing to do really but drop into the moment sensorially, and he did. With surprising ease, the tension and holding in his muscles gave way to a soft childlike quality.

Then something magical happened. A deep, delightful sound cascaded out of Michael. He laughed the completely infectious laugh of abandoned delight and pleasure. We all joined in and surrendered together to the moment. There was nowhere else to go.

"This is 'it'! This is the feeling I wanted to feel." Michael said in a low, round voice that came out of his belly.

Michael was having the experience of the Beloved that Rumi describes, where the heart opens and the Spirit enters. He was joined with himself, body and soul. He was joined with the group, with the whole gestalt, and all was right with the world. He was bathing in a state of true essence.

CHAPTER 12

Epilogue

Today, like every other day, we wake up empty and
frightened
Don't open the door to the study and begin reading.
Take down a musical instrument.

Let the beauty we love be what we do.
There are hundreds of ways to kneel and kiss the
ground.

— RUMI

Opening our senses means opening to the world and all that is.

Our senses connect us to our ancestors.

Our senses are the direct voice of our DNA.

Our senses allow us to see, hear, smell, taste, and feel what it means to be alive in the world right now.

An open and impartial awareness allows us to listen to the messages of our senses, the wisdom of the body, and live in the world with balance, appreciation, and grace.

The subtitle of this book is "The Art and Practice of Living in Your Body." A well-tuned body combined with fair-witness consciousness is the simple formula for developing and maintaining a state of impartial and open awareness. But be forewarned: This is not a path you can walk down in a day. Awareness is an art, and it is a practice.

It takes commitment, passion, inspiration, courage, and discipline to transform the human instrument into a Stradivarius.

May you find the courage it takes to enjoy both the instrument and the symphony.

Organizations of Interest

Lomi School
Lomi Community Clinic, 600 B Street, Santa Rosa, CA, 95401.
Phone: (707) 579-0465
E-mail: LomiSchool@aol.com

Feldenkrais Guild
3611 Southwest Hood Avenue, Suite 100, Portland, OR 97201.
Phone: (800) 775-2118
E-mail: guild@feldenkrais.com
Internet: www.feldenkrais.com

Naropa University
2130 Arapahoe Avenue, Boulder, CO 80302.
Phone: (303) 444-0202
Fax: (303) 444-0410
E-mail: info@naropa.edu
Internet: http://www.naropa.edu

Aikido of Tamalpais
76 East Blithedale Avenue, Mill Valley, CA 94941.
Phone: (415) 383-9474
E-mail: info@tam-aikido.org

United States Association of Body-Psychotherapy
7831 Woodmont Ave., PMB 294, Bethesda, MD 20814.
Phone: (202) 466-1619
E-mail: USABP@usabp.org

Spirit Rock Meditation Center
P.O. Box 169, Woodacre, CA 94973.
Phone: 415-488-0164
Fax: 415-488-0170
E-mail: SRMC@spiritrock.org
Internet: http://www.spiritrock.org

Esalen Institute
Highway 1, Big Sur, CA 93920-9616.
Phone: 831-667-3000
Fax: 831-667-2724
E-mail: info@esalen.org
Internet: http://www.esalen.org

CIIS (California Institute of Integral Studies)
1453 Mission Street, San Francisco, CA 94103.
Phone: 415-575-6100
Fax: 415-575-1264
E-mail: info@ciis.edu
Internet: http://www.ciis.edu

Barks, Coleman and Michael Green. *The Illuminated Rumi*. Broadway Books, 1997.

Berman, Morris. *Coming to Our Senses: Body and Spirit in the Hidden History of the West*. Simon & Schuster, 1989.

De Becker, Gavin. *The Gift of Fear: Survival Signals That Protect Us from Violence*. Little, Brown & Company, 1997.

Eisler, Riane. *Sacred Pleasure, Sex, Myth and the Politics of the Body—New Paths to Power and Love*. HarperSanFrancisco, 1996.

Feldenkrais, Moshe. *Awareness Through Movement: Health Exercises for Personal Growth*. Harper & Row, 1977.

Goldstein, Joseph and Jack Kornfield. *Seeking the Heart of Wisdom: The Path of Insight Meditation*. Shambala, 1987.

Heckler, Richard Strozzi. *The Anatomy of Change: East/West Approaches to Body/Mind Therapy*. North Atlantic Books, 1993.

Horney, Karen. *Our Inner Conflicts: A Constructive Theory of Neurosis*. W. W. Norton & Company, 1945.

Johnson, Don Hanlon. *Groundworks: Narratives of Embodiment*. North Atlantic Books, 1997.

Lowen, Alexander. *The Language of the Body*. Collier Books, 1958.

Miller, Alice. *Thou Shalt Not Be Aware: Society's Betrayal of the Child*. A Meridian Book, 1990.

Montagu, Ashley. *Touching: The Human Significance of the Skin*. Harper & Row, 1986

Napier, Augustus Y. and Carl Whitaker. *The Family Crucible: The Intense Experience of Family Therapy*. Harper Perennial, 1978.

Naranjo, Claudio. *Character and Neurosis: An Integrative View*. Gateways/IDHHB, Inc., 1994.

———*Gestalt Therapy: The Attitude & Practice of an Atheoretical Experientialism*. Gateways/IDHHB, Inc., 1993.

Palmer, Helen. *The Enneagram: The Definitive Guide to the Ancient System for Understanding Yourself and the Others in Your Life*. Harper & Row, 1988.

Palmer, Wendy. *The Intuitive Body: Aikido as a Clairsentient Practice*. North Atlantic Books, 1994.

Perls, Frederick S. *Gestalt Therapy Verbatim*. Gestalt Journal Press, 1992.

Reich, Wilhelm. *The Function of the Orgasm*. Noonday Press, 1986.

Sapolsky, Robert M. *Why Zebras Don't Get Ulcers: A Guide to Stress, Stress Related Diseases, and Coping*. W. H. Freeman and Company, 1998.

Ulysses Press Health Books

THE 7 HEALING CHAKRAS: UNLOCKING YOUR BODY'S ENERGY CENTERS
ISBN 1-56975-168-4, 240 pp, $14.95
Explores the essence of chakras, vortices of energy that connect the physical body with the spiritual.

THE ANCIENT AND HEALING ART OF AROMATHERAPY
ISBN 1-56975-094-7, 96 pp, $14.95
Discusses the benefits and history of aromatherapy.

THE ANCIENT AND HEALING ART OF CHINESE HERBALISM
ISBN 1-56975-139-0, 96 pp, $14.95
Offers a beautifully illustrated history and demonstrates the uses of Chinese herbalism.

HEALING REIKI: REUNITE MIND, BODY AND SPIRIT
WITH HEALING ENERGY
ISBN 1-56975-162-5, 128 pp, $16.95
Examines the meaning, attitudes and history of Reiki while providing practical tips for receiving and giving this universal life energy.

KNOW YOUR BODY: THE ATLAS OF ANATOMY
2nd edition, ISBN 1-56975-166-8, 160 pp, $14.95
Provides a a comprehensive, full-color guide to the human body.

MOOD FOODS
ISBN 1-56975-023-8, 192 pp, $11.95
Shows how the foods you eat influence your emotions and behavior.

NEW AGAIN!: THE 28-DAY DETOX PLAN FOR BODY AND SOUL
ISBN 1-56975-190-0, 128 pp, $16.95
Allows you to free your body and mind from toxins and live a healthy and balanced life.

SEX HERBS: NATURE'S SEXUAL ENHANCERS FOR MEN AND WOMEN
ISBN 1-56975-185-4, 328 pp, $14.95
Presents detailed descriptions of safe, natural products that boost sexual desire and pleasure.

YOUR NATURAL PREGNANCY: A GUIDE TO COMPLEMENTARY THERAPIES
ISBN 1-56975-059-9, 240 pp, $16.95
Details alternative therapies ranging from aromatherapy to yoga that can benefit pregnant women.

———

To order these books call 800-377-2542 or 510-601-8301, fax 510-601-8307; visit our website at www.ulyssespress.com; or write to Ulysses Press, P.O. Box 3440, Berkeley, CA 94703-3440. All retail orders are shipped free of charge. California residents must include sales tax. Allow two to three weeks for delivery.